Life will never be the same again

Life will never be the same again

Learning to be a first-time parent

A review of antenatal and postnatal health education

Gill Combes
Anne Schonveld

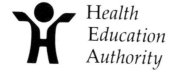

*Health
Education
Authority*

ISBN 1 85448 36 1 7

© Health Education Authority, 1992
Hamilton House
Mabledon Place
London WC1H 9TX

Printed and bound in Great Britain by
Biddles Ltd, Guildford and King's Lynn

Contents

Acknowledgements

This review was commissioned and funded by the Health Education Authority and carried out by the Community Education Development Centre, Coventry.

Thanks are due to all the parents who took part in the research detailed in Section 3, for sharing their views and experiences with us so openly. The parents were recruited to discussion groups by Quality Fieldwork of Sutton Coldfield, West Midlands.

Useful comments and support for this work were given by:

Dorit Braun   Community Education Development Centre
Karen Ford   Health Education Authority
Christine McGuire   Health Education Authority
and, at a later stage, by:
Kathy Elliott   Health Education Authority

The views expressed in this publication are those of the authors and do not necessarily reflect the views or policies of the Health Education Authority or the Community Education Development Centre.

Foreword

The Health Education Authority (HEA) is a special health authority within the National Health Service. Its mission is to ensure that 'by the year 2000, the people of England are more knowledgeable, better motivated and more able to acquire and maintain good health'.

This research report is the first stage of a long-term project by the HEA to develop innovative ways of supporting new parents. It is a key area in health education: each year almost 300,000 women (1) give birth to a child for the first time and go through the experience of becoming a parent. A further 400,000 women give birth to a child for the second time or more.

For first-time parents in particular, this is often a time of uncertainty and adjustment, when both women and their partners experience changes in their physical and emotional health, in their personal and social relationships and in their lifestyles, finances and aspirations. Not surprisingly, women and, increasingly, men are often receptive to health messages and interested in information, advice and shared experiences which can help them to adjust to these life changes. It offers an opportunity to make positive changes in their lifestyle which may be long-lasting and have benefits to health generally.

This is also a time when women in particular have regular contact with health professionals in a variety of hospital and community settings – health professionals who are in a position to offer support, information and advice on a broad range of health-related issues relevant to these life changes. This includes health education about pregnancy, birth and childcare, and the health and well-being of the parents themselves. The HEA has encountered a constant demand from health professionals for more and better materials with which to support parents at this time and we needed to look at in closer detail.

Set against this there are other factors which influence parent education today: there is a large number of other sources of advice and information for parents, family and friends and the media; there is unequal use of the health services by different socio-economic and racial groups, and changes in health-service funding and priorities which are influencing the opportunities and resourcing of parent education.

The research published here sets the scene. It reviews current provision from the perspective of both parents and professionals. It seeks to identify the experiences and needs of those who become parents for the first time, and to evaluate parents' views about the kinds of parent education they have experienced. It also seeks to assess the views of health professionals and those in voluntary agencies who work on parent education, to identify successes and difficulties and particularly to evaluate its effectiveness as a means of health education.

The next phase will see this research distilled into a range of parent education materials capable of working in a variety of settings, with many different groups – both professional and lay – alongside two of the HEA's most successful and popular publications, *Pregnancy Book* and *Birth to five*. In working with Community Education Development Centre (CEDC) on this long-term project, the HEA believes that an exciting, flexible and innovative way forward for parent education, to support subsequent generations of parents, will be developed.

Karen Ford
Christine McGuire
Health Education Authority
January 1992

(1) In 1990, the number of first births in England was 298 695 (OPCS, 1991.)

Summary

Parent education is an important area of work for many health professionals who are involved in the care and support of families that are expecting a baby or have recently had a baby. This review sets out to explore how parent education currently works in practice, from the perspective of both parents and professionals, and identifies ways in which it could become more effective. Whilst the focus is on health professionals and the health service, the review does include parent education within voluntary organizations, and should be relevant to all practitioners irrespective of the sector in which they work.

This review summarizes information and research from three sources: an overview of literature published in this country over the last 10 years; a small piece of qualitative research with parents and prospective parents; and a series of interviews with professionals and professional organizations. It considers parent education during antenatal and postnatal periods; this happens on a one-to-one basis and in groups, both informally and formally, and both between parents and professionals and amongst parents themselves. The review is based around three key questions:

- What needs do parents have for education?
- How are these needs being met? Are they being met appropriately and effectively?
- Is parent education equally accessible and appropriate to all?

The main findings were:

- Needs and provision are mismatched
- Certain parents are missing out
- Education in care settings is underestimated
- Men are missing out
- There is a narrow focus
- Aims are unclear
- Educational quality is poor
- Management support is lacking

Needs and provision are mismatched

In antenatal classes the focus of provision leaves relatively little time for questions, discussion or more formal education within antenatal care. This means that the needs in the first and second trimester of pregnancy are often poorly met, or met too late in the third trimester. This is particularly so for health and lifestyle issues such as diet, smoking and alcohol use, where changes in behaviour in early pregnancy can influence both maternal and child health.

The focus of postnatal provision is on one-to-one education and support, with relatively poor provision of postnatal groups. Within hospitals, many women's needs immediately after the birth are not met because of pressures of ward organization and ethos.

Parents who miss out

Attendance at antenatal classes and postnatal groups is largely by White, middle-class educated women. Less than half of all pregnant women attend any classes, and even fewer attend most or all sessions. Certain groups of parents are missing out on parent education in groups – particularly those who are young, single, working-class or from an ethnic minority group. These are also the women who have greater needs by virtue of having poorer levels of existing information, poorer access to health services and a greater chance of ill health for both mother and baby.

Underestimating education in care settings

Despite the high take-up of antenatal and postnatal care, by all groups of women (including those unlikely to attend classes), health professionals tend not to give much time to education within care settings. Certain aspects of care also mitigate against many women asking questions and feeling able to discuss anxieties or problems. A common focus within care on medical and physical health may also mean that women's social and emotional health needs go unmet.

Men miss out

Women are almost universally the target group for parent education despite the ever-increasing recognition of the important role men play as parents and in family life. Men are largely excluded from antenatal and postnatal classes, which are still not universally offered to men, and which may not meet their needs.

Professionals express ambivalence and uncertainty about addressing men's needs as parents.

A narrow focus

Overall, much parent education focuses on giving information on a narrow range of medical and physical health issues. Social, emotional and psychological aspects of parent education are less well recognized by parent educators and less often addressed in both care and group settings.

Unclear aims

A plethora of aims exists for parent education, ranging from influencing health in pregnancy and making labour easier, to teaching parenting skills, increasing parents' confidence in their own abilities and developing support networks among parents. This diversity of aims is reflected in the detail of practice and in approaches to evaluation. Overall, there is a lack of clarity about what parent education might be expected to achieve.

Poor educational quality

Both parents and professionals express concerns about the effectiveness of parent education. For parents, information and knowledge needs are generally acknowledged and addressed by health professionals, whilst broader social and emotional needs often go unmet. For professionals, there is an awareness that the way classes, groups or care settings are organized often reduces educational effectiveness.

Lack of management support

As an area of professional practice, parent education generally has poor managerial support, in relation to the key areas of resourcing, training and development. Attempts to improve practice by practitioners have often floundered as a result, and significant improvements to practice are unlikely to happen without managerial support.

Recommendations

The report makes seven key recommendations.

1. Improve educational quality

The aim of parent education should be primarily educational and therefore not prescriptive about health or behavioural outcomes. There is a need to give equal emphasis to knowledge, skills, feelings and attitudes, and to work to the agendas of both parents and health professionals. Active participation in learning needs to be encouraged so that parents can review their own ideas and knowledge, learn from one another, and apply information to their own circumstances. The information base for parent education needs to develop greater sensitivity to the individual social, cultural, economic and family backgrounds of parents.

2. Recognize individual needs

Parent education needs to develop greater sensitivity to the individual needs of parents. A particularly important part of this is recognizing the restricted choices that some parents face, and recognizing that for these parents education plays a limited part in enabling change. For parents in poverty or experiencing particular disadvantages, support will be an inextricable part of education. Professionals should be encouraged to recognize how support increases the effectiveness of education, and how education can itself be supportive through the use of peer learning and an open-ended approach.

3. Take a broad focus

Parent education should be relevant to the concerns and lives of parents as they go through pregnancy, labour and the early months of parenting. Greater emphasis needs to be given to the psychological, emotional and social aspects of parents' experiences. A realistic approach means that education should cover difficult as well as positive experiences and issues, and particularly help to create realistic expectations of labour and of parenting. The amount of time generally given to breathing and relaxation in antenatal classes should be reduced in proportion to its significance within the whole experience of becoming a parent, thus releasing time for the consideration of other issues.

4. Provide education at the time of need

During pregnancy parents should have opportunities for education at the time of need, appropriate to their stage of pregnancy. Greater emphasis needs to be given to education in the second and especially the first trimester, when the health of the mother can have some influence on the health of the developing baby. Postnatally, more attention could be given to the provision of support groups during the first 6 weeks, and after the first 4 or 5 months.

5. Maximize the use of existing opportunities

Many opportunities for parent education go unnoticed or underused because of focusing attention on antenatal classes. In practice, many different health professionals are in regular contact with a woman during pregnancy and the early months of parenting, and each have a part to play in both education and support. Particular attention should be paid to how routine antenatal and postnatal clinic care can be organized so that parents have more opportunities to ask questions, discuss anxieties and choices, and have more informal contact with other parents who can provide support and share experiences.

In view of the documented fact that the uptake of routine care is far greater than for groups both antenatally and postnatally, priority should be given to increasing the effectiveness of the existing opportunities provided during routine care, rather than attempting to expand the provision of groups. An exception to this is the need for specially targeted antenatal classes for groups considered to either have special needs or reduced access to health services (the ethnic minority and young women in particular). Specially targeted classes for these groups may often provide unique opportunities for education not readily available elsewhere.

Within the health service, recognition is needed of the important part already played by other statutory services and voluntary organizations.

6. Provide for fathers and partners

There is an urgent need to consider how parent education can provide for the needs and wishes of fathers and partners. At present, they have virtually no involvement in routine antenatal or postnatal care and only peripheral involvement in postnatal hospital care. Their main access to parent education is through antenatal classes, which are still not generally on offer to all fathers and partners. In the short term, there is a need to extend antenatal class access to as many fathers and partners as possible, and encourage health professionals to consider how, in the longer term, their needs can be met through other health service avenues.

7. A key role for management

Managers have a central and key role to play in supporting the development of parent education practice. They are in a position to address a number of linked factors, for instance, staffing, resourcing, training and the status of parent education, which currently stifle the development of practice in many areas.

Managers should take responsibility for reviewing practice in their local area in order to identify barriers to progress, to review targets for improvement, and to support practitioners in the implementation of change. Managers should have the dual aim of firstly improving parents' access to quality parent education, and secondly making parent education a more satisfying area of work for health professionals.

The review concludes with key questions for the development of practice in a local area. It also outlines the contribution which the development of resources and training could make to future practice.

Section 1: Introduction and Background

1.1 Scope of the review

The overall purpose of this review is to describe and analyse the current provision of parent education, both antenatally and postnatally, in Britain. It has a particular emphasis on evaluating the effectiveness of this provision and discussing ways in which both effective practice could be extended and built on, and gaps could be filled. Whilst its primary aim is to aid the future planning and development of work on parent education by the Health Education Authority, it is hoped that the review will also be relevant and interesting to both practitioners and managers.

1.2 Methods

This review draws together information from three sources.

1. A review of the literature

Since the literature on this topic is quite considerable (involving for this review a trawl of over 200 books, reports and articles), the review has been largely restricted to the period January 1980–March 1991, and to work undertaken in the United Kingdom. The only exceptions to these limits are where earlier work or overseas work makes a unique or particularly interesting contribution to the literature. The majority of this literature is on antenatal classes, with much less having been uncovered on education within antenatal care or in the postnatal period.

2. Research with parents

A small piece of qualitative research was undertaken with groups of pregnant women and first-time mothers to explore their experiences of pregnancy and on becoming a parent. Structured discussion groups with parents from a range of social, economic and racial backgrounds, were set up in rural, suburban and urban locations. The aim of this research was to help provide a framework based on the experiences and views of parents, within which current practice could be evaluated. Further details of the methods used and the results of this research are detailed in Section 3 of this report.

3. Interviews and discussions with professionals

In the period February–June 1991, interviews were conducted with 18 professionals and discussions held with two multi-professional groups involved in parent education. The purpose of these interviews was to consult key people and organizations in the field about issues for parent education now and in the future. A list of the people interviewed is given in Appendix 1. Themes from these interviews and discussions appear at relevant places throughout the report.

1.3 Evaluation criteria

This review covers a considerable volume of literature and research on parent education. In order to assess the effectiveness of parent education, four key criteria are used. Parent education should be:

- accessible to a reasonable proportion of parents
- considered useful by parents themselves
- be considered by health professionals as a useful and satisfying area of work
- be able to demonstrate tangible outcomes which are of value.

As for any evaluation, effectiveness can be judged on many different criteria which may be valued differently by different people. In recognition of this, the review which follows presents the evidence separately from a discussion of its significance and an assessment of its effectiveness. The evidence which is presented falls into four categories which broadly reflect the above criteria.

- Uptake studies – who has access to and takes up parent education and in which settings; who does not and the reasons for this.
- Consumer surveys – what parents feel about parent education. The relatively large number of consumer surveys undertaken in the past decade have tended to focus on antenatal classes.
- Professionals' views – how they feel about parent education, successes and blocks to its implementation. In contrast to consumer surveys, there has been very little research in this area. The review therefore relies quite heavily on the views of the professionals interviewed especially for this work.
- Outcome studies – changes which can be measured as a result of parent education, and objective evidence that it works, drawing on a series of about twenty research studies which have attempted to identify and quantify outcomes.

The relative merits and drawbacks of the above kinds of evidence are discussed briefly in Appendix 2.

Section 2: Parent education today

2.1 A brief history of parent education

The beginnings of parent education in this country can be traced to the second half of the nineteenth century, as part of an increasing concern for public health. In 1862 a scheme was set up in Manchester to offer advice on the care and health of children through house-to-house visits made by experienced mothers (Williams and Booth, 1985), and soon other towns followed by employing women as 'health visitors'. At the turn of the century the Boer War drew attention to the poor physical health of young men and this led to recommendations in the 1904 report of the Interdepartmental Committee on the Physical Deterioration of the Population (Tew, 1990) which included the education of mothers. In her review of the history of maternity care Tew notes that there followed a number of advisory circulars from the Local Government Board on treatment and medical advice for pregnant women. After the Ministry of Health was set up in 1919, a series of reports investigated various aspects of maternal and child health, and these included recommendations for widespread propaganda directed at women in order to convince them of the importance of their own health during pregnancy and their child-bearing years (Tew, 1990).

By the 1940s there was much advice available to the pregnant woman about self-care and health, clothing, preparation of the layette and the role of fathers (Sadler, 1988). However it was not until some years after the establishment of the National Health Service (NHS) in 1948, that formal antenatal classes began to be provided. The transfer of local authority, community-based antenatal clinics to the NHS, also led to an increasing medicalization of the care of pregnant women, and a transfer of much of their care from health visitors and midwives to general practitioners and obstetricians (Sadler, 1988). There followed three influential reports over a 20-year period which recommended increasingly that hospital was the safest place to give birth, whilst discouraging the once common practice of home delivery (see Cranbrook Committee, 1959, Peel Committee, 1970, and Short report, 1980 all cited in Tew, 1990).

Increases in hospital deliveries were paralleled by increased intervention in labour through techniques such as induction, foetal monitoring and drug use for pain relief (Gillet, 1985). Some authors point to this increasing medicalization of labour in the 1950s, 1960s, 1970s, as the main reason for increasing the provision of formal antenatal classes (for example, Gillet, 1985). The main purpose of these classes was seen as preparing women for a compliant and satisfactory hospital delivery. Other authors highlight post-war social changes such as increased geographical mobility and the demise of extended family structures (for example, Lindell, 1988). These changes are seen to have created a need for parent education, which had previously been met by immediate family and friends.

More recently, the recognition of child abuse as a significant problem has focused attention on the ways in which parents can and should be prepared for and supported in their parenting role. Parent education in the immediate antenatal and postnatal period can be seen as having an important part to play in developing realistic expectations of and skills for parenting (for example, Jamieson, 1986).

Post-war antenatal education

In parallel with the post-war trend towards the hospitalization and medicalization of pregnancy and labour, alternative thinking was developing on natural childbirth which subsequently had a strong influence on the content and approach of much antenatal education.

The first and probably most influential of these alternatives was put forward by Grantly Dick-Read, in 1944 (first edition). He maintained that childbirth is a natural physiological process which should not cause pain. However, anxieties and fears arising from cultural expectations cause tensions in the mind and body, and thus make labour a painful experience for many women. His promotion of pain-free labour through the use of the techniques of deep breathing and relaxation, and psychological and emotional preparation for birth, are still in evidence within most, if not all, NHS antenatal classes, and in the work of voluntary organizations such as the National Childbirth Trust (NCT).

A second school of thought, developed around the same time, promoted pain relief through psychoprophylaxis in which the reflex actions of the body are re-conditioned, so that labour sensations from the uterus are not perceived by the brain to be painful. This is achieved by educating women to believe that childbirth is not naturally painful, and by using special kinds of breathing and self-massage to block painful sensations (Williams and Booth, 1985). Psychoprophylaxis was originally developed in Russia, and grew out of Pavlov's ideas on conditioning, and observations of the value of hypnosis during childbirth. These ideas were developed further in France in the 1950s by Fernand Lamaze, who promoted different kinds of breathing and relaxation for the different stages of labour.

More recently, the active birth movement has promoted a move away from the rigid breathing patterns and mind-blocking techniques of psychoprophylaxis. Active birth stresses the importance of behaving instinctively, and of women being able to move about and find their own best positions for labour (Williams and Booth, 1985).

2.2   Education within antenatal care

The usual process of antenatal care offers a range of opportunities for one-to-one education on both a formal and informal basis. This starts for most women with the first contact, for confirmation of pregnancy, with the general practitioner (GP) or at a well woman or family planning clinic. At this point a woman may be given information or advice about health during pregnancy, and about the kind of antenatal care and education she may expect to receive from the health service. The GP refers each pregnant woman to an antenatal clinic which may be at the local hospital, at a separate community clinic or at the GP's own surgery. The first visit to the antenatal clinic, known as the booking visit, takes place from 12 weeks onwards, depending on how far into a pregnancy a woman is on the first visit to her GP and the speed and efficiency of the referral system. The booking visit is seen as a particularly important occasion during which a lot of information is gathered about a pregnant woman, and when her future care and delivery start to be planned. Subsequent clinic visits are offered throughout pregnancy, and are primarily times when the health of the mother and baby are monitored.

At some clinics women may have the opportunity to see a specialist such as a dietician or a welfare rights adviser. Otherwise, education takes place during the course of routine checks and screening, and on a one-to-one basis with a number of different health professionals, including consultant gynaecologists, GPs, midwives and health visitors. Their overall aim is to provide information and advice appropriate to the stage of the pregnancy and to respond to the individual needs and concerns of the women in their care. A wide range of health education literature is available to supplement and support this one-to-one education, most notably the *Pregnancy Book* (Health Education Authority, 1984) which is currently given free to all first-time pregnant women. In many areas, women may also receive one or more antenatal home visits from a community midwife and/or health visitor, which are intended to provide opportunities for both education and support. Most commonly, these home visits take place during the second half of pregnancy.

Overall, antenatal care provides regular contact between pregnant women and health professionals during which health issues are frequently discussed on a one-to-one basis. This happens in a planned way through the use of checklists, tests and records at different stages of pregnancy, and opportunistically in response to the concerns and questions of the pregnant woman.

2.3 Antenatal Classes

Antenatal classes provide the main formal educational opportunity for groups of pregnant women. They are usually offered for women to take up during the last trimester of pregnancy, from 26–28 weeks' confinement onwards. There is usually a set number of meetings, often between six and eight in total. They are held in community and/or hospital settings and run by a midwife and/or health visitor, often with additional input from an obstetric physiotherapist. Antenatal classes are generally designed to cover the following areas: health during pregnancy; labour; delivery and hospital procedures; learning relaxation and breathing techniques for use in labour; basic parenting and childcare. The exact content and balance of classes differs widely, as do the teaching methods and approaches used. However, it is common for between one third and one half of the time in each class to be taken up with exercises and relaxation/breathing techniques.

It is apparent from the literature that many district health authorities offer a range of antenatal classes, taking place in different locations and at different times during the day, sometimes including the evening. Some classes may be open to women only and some to women and fathers/partners/friends. As a minimum, fathers/partners/friends are usually invited to attend a special session and to join the labour ward visit.

In some areas there may be at least one of three kinds of additional antenatal class: preconception counselling, early pregnancy classes and aquanatal classes.

Outside of the health service, a national network of local antenatal classes is run by the National Childbirth Trust. These are self-financing and therefore run on a fee-paying basis. Similar topics are considered to those in many health service classes, with a particularly strong emphasis on:

- Sharing ideas and experiences in a group
- Encouraging women and their partners to identify and work for the kind of birth they would like
- Techniques for pain reduction

Whilst the majority of women attending and running NCT classes tend to be from middle-class backgrounds, the organization is increasingly trying to find ways of extending its work to include groups such as young women, single parents and ethnic minorities (NCT, 1991).

In some parts of the country, the organization Active Birth also runs antenatal classes to support women who wish to have a birth based on the ideas and techniques of the active birth movement (Williams and Booth, 1985).

2.4 Postnatal education

Opportunities for postnatal education currently occur largely on a one-to-one basis as part of the postnatal care offered to women in hospital and in the community. In the period immediately following the birth of a baby, women receive advice and support from hospital midwives, which transfers to the community midwife on returning home from hospital. Subsequently, the health visitor is involved in support, education and child health surveillance, through home visits and the services of the child health clinic.

In some areas, postnatal education or support groups provide additional opportunities for group-based education, although the number of postnatal groups is far less than for antenatal groups. Voluntary organizations such as the National Childbirth Trust also organize postnatal groups, whilst organizations such as Exploring Parenthood, EPIC and Newpin offer more specialized courses and group education on various aspects of being a parent.

2.5 The aims of parent education

From the literature, it is possible to identify six key aims for parent education. These are:

- To influence positively the health behaviour of women during pregnancy, and as parents
- To prepare women for labour and to enable parents to have an easier and more satisfying delivery
- To help prepare parents for parenthood, and support them in their role as parents
- To develop social support networks among parents
- To promote the development of skilled, confident and informed parents
- To contribute to reducing low birth weight and perinatal mortality and morbidity

The emphasis given to each of these aims varies quite considerably in the literature. In the antenatal period, many practitioners give particular emphasis to influencing women's health and preparing them for labour. In the postnatal period, support for the parents' role and the development of social support networks have common emphasis. The overall aim, about which most authors agree, is that parent education should contribute to producing a healthy and happy pregnancy and a healthy baby (for example, Ho, 1985).

There are, however, a number of areas of debate within the literature, about certain aspects of the aims of parent education. These areas of debate, which will re-emerge at various points throughout the review, can be summarized as follows:

- How far parents can be prepared in advance for their parental role, particularly in the antenatal period (Perkins, 1979).
- How far parent education can influence parenting, and what constitutes 'good' parenting (Perkins and Morris, 1981).

- Whether parents should be prepared for the realities of the health care system or educated to actively participate in it to achieve their personal choices, particularly about childbirth (Katona, 1981; Taylor, 1985; Lindell, 1988).
- How far parent education should be 'consumer' led, meeting parents' needs and concerns, and how far health professionals should direct its content (Taylor, 1985; Lindell, 1988).
- How far parent education is about education or about outcomes relating to health (Butler, 1985).
- How far work on parents' personal development can contribute to the goals of healthier and happier parents (Dunwoody and Watters, 1990; Jeffs, 1990).
- Whether parent education is primarily about women and babies or about the family as a whole (Perkins, 1979).

Section 3: Becoming a parent – the views of pregnant women and new parents

3.1 Introduction

As part of this review on parent education in England a small piece of research into the experiences of new parents was commissioned. The remit of the research was purposely very broad: to discuss with groups of pregnant women and first-time parents their experiences, feelings and concerns about becoming a parent. It was hoped that this research would help to identify needs of relevance to parent education: What are parents' needs? Who meets them and how? What role do health services and health professionals play in meeting these needs? What improvements could be made?

This section summarizes the issues raised by groups of parents and prospective parents taking part in discussion groups in the West Midlands in the spring of 1991. The research was small-scale, qualitative and open-ended in nature. It provides a picture of the experiences and concerns of a small number of parents, and suggests pointers for improving practice. It is intended to stimulate and provoke questions, rather than provide a detailed view of a representative group of parents. It is also intended to help anchor this review of parent education in the lives of parents themselves.

3.2 Approach and methods

The research took as its main focus the experiences of women. As a small-scale piece of research, it was not possible to target both men and women. The aims of the research were to explore with pregnant women and first-time mothers:

- their experiences during pregnancy
- their experiences during the first months of parenting

Small groups of up to ten parents were invited to take part in a discussion session on becoming a parent. A total of 58 parents took part in nine different discussion groups. One of these groups was for men only, and who were partners of pregnant women. The remaining groups were of pregnant women or first-time mothers. Full details of the ways in which the groups were convened and of the methods used are given in Appendix 3.

3.3 Pregnancy

1. Likes and dislikes of pregnancy

What most women liked about pregnancy

Most of the women talked of feeling more important and special when they were visibly pregnant. One said:

> I felt very important, you know – the doctors and nurses all treated you as if you were very important. After the baby came along that side changed – then it was going from being the most important person to your husband and family and everybody, to 'How old's the baby?' and 'How are you, by the way?' You know, I enjoyed all the fuss and that – it was good.

They commented on how people generally showed them consideration and were interested in them. They enjoyed the attention and cosseting, although for some this became overwhelming when they were 'made to feel like an invalid' or 'wrapped in cotton wool', or 'treated like a mental defective'.

Some commented that they felt healthier when pregnant and how their hair and skin improved. They welcomed the cessation of periods and not needing to worry about contraception. One woman commented on the joy of being pregnant after waiting so long to conceive and many women talked about their excitement at seeing the scan, the sense of the baby being real, and delight at feeling the baby kick. As one woman said:

> I felt safe because the baby was kicking.

Some were enjoying buying baby clothes and equipment, and decorating the house or baby's room in preparation. For some, leaving work had been a relief and for others it had meant boredom and loneliness. One woman told about being honest at an interview about her pregnancy and feeling sure that this was why she didn't get the job. Most women mentioned reading books about the development of the foetus and enjoying looking at the diagrams and pictures of the baby developing.

What women disliked about pregnancy

This was generally discussed much more than what was liked about pregnancy. Almost all the women interviewed mentioned the physical changes and sensations: morning sickness, varicose veins and swollen legs, backache and tiredness. They also talked about being emotionally changeable and weepy.

Some women talked of feeling less attractive and of not being able to find or afford to buy attractive maternity clothes. They commented on stretch marks and feeling heavy and cumbersome. Some found it difficult to drive in later pregnancy and to wear a seat belt.

In the early months, before women had let it be generally known that they were pregnant, some felt criticized for taking time off work when they felt unwell, and that other people were not sympathetic to their mood changes and vulnerability. Some commented on how people in the street, particularly men, stared at them when they were more visibly pregnant.

Some talked of feeling guilty at being less than ecstatic about being pregnant:

> You're supposed to feel great. Just because I'm pregnant doesn't mean to say I have to be happy about it.

One woman told of her fantasy about being pregnant and her enjoyment of seeing pregnant women and how this had changed. She wasn't enjoying pregnancy 'for real' and was much more scared than she had anticipated.

They also commented on how aware they were becoming of facilities for babies in public places, and access to shops and lifts.

> Our shopping centre has a beautiful baby room, and it's on the third floor up and the lift is broken. You have to leave the prams and everything at the bottom and go up the escalator with the baby and come down for the changing stuff. And there's masses of empty space downstairs – but they put it on the third floor.

Some women said they worried about how a baby would change their relationship with their partners. For some, the responsibility of a dependent baby weighed heavily on their minds, as did the anticipated loss of freedom and independence. For those living with parents there was the problem of finding accommodation. Some said that friends who were not pregnant or parents had withdrawn, as if they now had less in common.

When talking about their expectations of being a first time parent most women mentioned tiredness and sleeplessness as a main worry. They also talked of how anxious they felt about coping on their own with a small baby. Some feared tiredness and stress might lead to arguments within the relationship and some were worried that they wouldn't have enough patience with a crying baby. Most mentioned their desire for postnatal support groups for 'when the problems really start'. Some were already anticipating the conflict of staying at home with the baby and returning to work.

2. Experiences, feelings and concerns at the different stages of pregnancy

A number of recurring themes came through from the groups, about what it is commonly like to be pregnant, at the different stages of pregnancy. These are summarized in Table 1.

Table 1: Women's experiences, feelings and concerns at the different stages of pregnancy

0–3 months	• Ambivalent feelings about being pregnant and the need for opportunities to discuss these
	• Physical complaints – tiredness, morning sickness
	• Feelings of panic and anxiety about labour and being a parent
	• Worrying about the baby's health and about miscarriage
	• Anxieties about diet and receiving conflicting advice about diet
	• Enjoying the extra attention and care
3–6 months	• Enjoying the baby kick and feeling more aware of it
	• Feeling safer from the threat of miscarriage
	• Difficulties with finding clothes
	• Feeling unattractive
6–9 months	• Becoming tired of working
	• Increased anxiety about labour and birth
	• Enjoying buying things for the baby and getting ready for its arrival
	• Having to cope with hearing other people's experiences
	• Difficulties with being comfortable and sleeping
	• Body image – worrying about getting shape back
	• Worries about the birth

3. Health issues and relationships with health professionals

Early pregnancy

For many women their first experience of health care in pregnancy was the visit to the GP for the results of the pregnancy test. Many women felt 'let down' at this point with little opportunity to discuss how they felt about being pregnant. Some single women felt their doctor assumed the pregnancy was a mistake and one was offered termination, whilst married women thought their doctors often assumed they would be happy about the pregnancy. Doctors were sometimes lacking in understanding about the difficulties of getting time off work for appointments, and were less than sensitive about internal examinations.

Many women commented on the lack of information about diet and foods to avoid in early pregnancy, and some commented on conflicting advice which left them feeling confused and unsure. One woman said:

My doctor just told me about liver and cream cheese

and later she telephoned to check:

The receptionist wandered off and then she says, 'oh yes that will be fine'.

Some women said they felt that the advice was given too late on in pregnancy, given the importance of health care in the early months. Women with particular conditions such as asthma worried about whether they would be able to take advantage of certain drugs in labour and most women were somewhat anxious about the effects of any medication during pregnancy. Overall, many women said that this was a time in their pregnancy when they would have welcomed more information, advice and support but weren't sure where to go or were not confident enough to ask.

Middle and late pregnancy

Many women complained of long waits at clinics and long journeys to hospital which were especially difficult for women who already had small children. When at the clinic, they talked of lack of time and opportunities to ask questions and discuss their feelings about their pregnancy.

Some mentioned information needs they had but hadn't expressed. Most wanted more information about Caesarian and forceps deliveries, induction and epidurals. They worried about labour, about how they would know it had started, how painful it would be and how long it would last. One woman felt that her questions had not been properly discussed. On her visit to the hospital she had said:

> I've got a few questions to ask and when can I ask them? Can I ask you now? Should I wait or is there somebody else? And I've got them written down – and she said 'well tell me a couple', and I told her and one of them was I'd like to have the choice of forceps and the vacuum thing – that I wanted the vacuum thing because I didn't fancy the forceps and she went straight down my throat . . . and she was really against me wanting to know anything and she said 'Don't worry about it, forget it all, leave it, you don't want to know'.

When she talked about the birth plan and wanting to put forward her thoughts, she was told 'the doctors know what they're doing – they know best – leave it to them'. She said she felt disappointed and surprised at that reaction.

Anxiety was expressed about waiting for test results and the numbers of tests that had to be taken. Most women worried about whether their baby would be all right.

> I had to have a blood test, and they phoned me up and said the results of that were low and there was a possibility she might be handicapped, so I had to wait to have that amniocentesis and you have to wait 3–5 weeks for the results and that was very stressful.

One woman told of waiting for test results:

> I had a letter come and I thought, oh God, it's from the hospital – but they told me I wouldn't get a letter so I was thinking I daren't open this letter, something is wrong.

Many women said they would prefer to be notified of test results automatically, even when they were negative, in order to put their minds at rest. Being told they would only hear if something was wrong was not enough, because there might have been a mistake somewhere along the line which they would never know about.

Some of the single women felt that they had been treated differently by the health professionals. In addition to the assumptions made by GPs (reported above), women felt the health professionals assumed they would not cope and maybe would not care so much about their pregnancy and their baby. They disliked these assumptions.

Antenatal classes

Most women who attended antenatal classes were positive about the experience but most bemoaned the lack of time to talk about individual concerns. Some women had missed the opportunity to get to classes through being hospitalized early or being delivered early. One woman who had been unaware of her pregnancy when she went into labour regretted that she had missed out on the preparatory stages and the anticipation of becoming a parent. Another had been unable to go to classes because her local ones were all full.

Women enjoyed the social contact with other women at the classes. Some felt that the breathing and relaxation exercises had helped their labour and most had enjoyed the visit to the labour ward. They had also found the videos useful. Some women felt that the information about where and when the classes were held was unclear and would have appreciated greater clarity and direction on this. One woman described a huge evening class she had gone to where she could hardly hear because of the numbers there. Most women preferred smaller groups.

Some women felt that 'difficult' topics, such as abnormal labour, were avoided or dealt with only briefly. They felt that the teachers tended to dismiss anxieties or negative feelings. Many women would have welcomed more information on Caesarian sections, epidurals and forceps deliveries.

A number of women commented on the pressure there was to breast-feed and that bottle feeding was given less time in the classes. They also mentioned that advice given in the classes was often different from advice from other health professionals.

In some classes, very little time had been given to considering what happens after the birth and how to cope with being a parent. For first-time mothers this was a common and important criticism. However, they did feel that they may not have been very open to these issues because they were so concerned with labour and the birth. A common suggestion was to have a new mother to visit the classes to talk about her experiences of being a parent.

Some women made an overall criticism of the classes that they focused too much on the baby and not enough on the feelings and experiences of the mother.

I felt I lost my identity – the baby was the only thing that mattered.

For some this was explained by the observation that the teacher was not a mother herself – an issue raised by most groups, generally as a criticism.

Finally, women who had had partners with them at classes expressed ambivalent feelings about how it had affected them. Some felt that having partners there meant they would worry and therefore be of less support. Others felt sensitive about discussing certain issues in front of men.

For those women who had not been to classes or were currently not going, most felt that they did not need to attend. They were happy with the information they already had, and many mentioned having found out a lot from friends and family. For single women in the urban groups, going to classes seemed to be equated with failing to cope. They felt confident about their pregnancies, and were particularly anxious to be seen to be coping well, especially as they knew health professionals were often very concerned about single parents.

3.4 Being a first-time parent

1. The early months

Most women felt that the tiredness was greater than they had anticipated. As one woman said:

> There should be some sort of instruction to tell you exactly what's involved because I don't think we do go into it – we just think of the baby – we don't think of afterwards.

They talked of the immense responsibility of a baby and felt panic-stricken at times, that it was a 'total nightmare'. Lack of freedom to go out spontaneously without relying on someone else to baby-sit had been difficult for some. Those who managed to get out in the early weeks often found they worried about the baby and were reluctant to go out for long. Some talked of being 'in chaos' and of how long it took to establish a routine. Many talked of their fears about cot deaths and of leaning over the cot to make sure the baby was breathing.

Some women talked about their body image and their feelings about the changes that had taken place, and of their partners' insensitivity about their changed shape. They talked of how it took longer to get back into their pre-pregnancy clothes than they had imagined.

Establishing breast-feeding, dealing with colic and crying seemed to be the main preoccupations. Some women spoke of their ambivalence about breast-feeding in public or in front of their relatives. One woman said she felt her child 'couldn't just have me for myself, all she wanted was the breast'. Several women expressed confusion at the advice given about breast-feeding. One mother said:

> I wanted to breast-feed and bottle-feed as well and they said no, you can't do the two – just do one. I didn't have enough milk you see, that's why it was taking so long – and they wouldn't let me go on to changing to the bottle. At about three months, he put on two ounces and he ended up in hospital. They told me to bottle-feed him – they really made me depressed.

Several women expressed sentiments along the lines of this mother:

> They tell you to breast-feed and don't explain it to you properly, you're always scared the baby's not putting weight on.

Women talked about conflicting advice from professionals leaving them feeling confused and uncertain. As one women said:

> You need continuity I think because when you're a first-time mum you are a bit anxious and you're made to feel a complete and utter idiot. Now I'm just getting on with it – and I think well if she's happy that's the main thing.

For many, going home with a new baby meant tensions with parents about looking after a new baby and who was in control. Some resented the way relatives, and particularly their mothers, interfered with their care of the baby and gave unwelcome advice. For some, the excitement of having the baby led to a feeling of 'just me and the baby' when they came home and of feeling 'dumped'. Some welcomed visitors but others felt intruded upon. Some resented that the focus was entirely on the baby and that they felt 'like a baby machine'. What many said they wanted most was peace, time with their baby and partner, and rest.

Some women also mentioned the need to talk about what the birth had been like.

2. From 4 months onwards

When talking about older babies (4 or 5 months) many mothers commented on their pleasure at seeing their babies progress and develop. As the babies slept better, the mothers were able to get more rest. They mentioned the difficulties of leaving their babies at this stage with other carers, as the bonding between mother and child grew.

As the baby developed many mothers commented on how they checked their development against books to see how they were progressing. Some said they felt these books were useful as rough guides, but worrying if taken too literally as babies develop at different paces.

Talking about older babies (6 or 7 months) many women commented on how exhausting it was watching them all the time to make sure they were safe. Their babies slept less in the daytime and therefore they had less time to catch up on their household jobs. Some had begun teething and so were sometimes wakeful at night. Many commented on the support they had received from their immediate families and partners, although some also expressed the fear of being overpowered with advice and losing the feeling of the baby being theirs.

The recurring themes from the groups about their experiences, feelings and concerns in the early months of being a first-time parent are summarized in Table 2.

Table 2: Women's experiences, feelings and concerns in the first months of parenting

0–3 months	• Experiencing differences between hospital and home, especially in the support provided
	• Fears of not coping, being disorganized
	• Lack of sleep, exhaustion
	• Lack of freedom and having to fit your own needs around those of the baby
	• Ambivalence about whether to work
	• Coping with relatives and family
	• Establishing breast-feeding
	• Conflicting advice about feeding and baby management from relatives and professionals
	• Anxieties about weight gain
	• Enjoying people's responses to the new baby
4–6 months	• Enjoying watching the baby develop
	• Baby becoming more demanding of attention
	• Trying to regain pre-pregnancy shape
	• Difficulties with weaning
7–9 months	• Enjoying the development of the baby
	• Baby becoming more active, so having little time for yourself
	• Teething causing disturbed sleep
	• Worrying and checking with books about the baby's development

3. Health issues and relationships with health professionals

In hospital

Many women shared their experiences of being in hospital and their confusion at the conflicting advice and practices. For Asian women there were the problems of language and for some, of diet and the isolation of not understanding hospital procedures. For some women there was a sense of not being regarded as an individual but just a body. One woman commented:

> There just don't seem to be enough people there, when you're in labour you're just attached to a machine and they just come in and they look at the machine and then they look at you and say 'Are you alright?' Some of them just walk in and look at the machine and walk out again.

Some women commented on the different practices in hospital and between hospitals.

> I found if you're in labour through the day they give you an epidural but when I went in it was two o'clock in the morning and they said the emergency doctor wouldn't come out – that was the reason why I couldn't have one.

For many women the experience of hospitals was confusing and depersonalising:

You just feel like a number, a piece of cattle.

Some women in hospital felt supported in their attempts to breast-feed, others didn't. Many commented that breast-feeding mothers got more attention than those who bottle-fed, and some felt guilty about their choice of feeding. Some enjoyed the privacy of single rooms and the extra attention from the nurses, and others felt deprived of the company of other women. Most women emphasized the need for time from sympathetic staff and the need to talk.

At home and at the clinic

Once home, most women were positive about the support they received from the midwife and health visitor, although a desire for more information emerged as to why health visitors and midwives 'do certain things to the baby'. One mother felt suspicious, after recent cases in the newspaper of bogus health professionals, about her baby being 'stripped off' and examined. Most were unsure about what a midwife/health visitor was entitled to do and what practices a mother could rightly object to.

Some women experienced feelings of being judged and monitored in their care of the baby, and as to their adequacy as mothers. One woman mentioned her fear that her health visitor had a 'little black book' where comments were written down, and fears were expressed about losing their children.

Some women expressed uncertainty about the different roles of midwives and health visitors. They also commented regretfully on the number of different professionals who had dealt with them during pregnancy, birth and aftercare, and many felt unable to establish a relationship because of these staff changes. Some had also felt the visits by midwife or health visitor to be intrusive and would have preferred to know when they were coming, rather than their just popping in. Some of the single women again said they felt they were being watched and that they needed to show they could cope. They often felt they had to do 'better' than mothers with a partner.

Conflicting advice from health professionals was a recurring issue particularly in relation to breast-feeding.

Some women also talked about anxiety about minor ailments and illnesses. They felt unsure about symptoms, and were not confident about when it was necessary to visit the GP or the clinic. For some, their experiences at the GP surgery undermined their confidence. They felt their worries were not taken seriously and that they were dismissed as 'fussing first-time mums'.

3.5 The additional groups

The discussions with fathers, second-time mothers and Asian women raised a number of important issues. These related directly to the experiences and concerns of these groups, and are reported in this section. Second-time mothers and the Asian women also said many things about pregnancy and being a parent which were similar to women in the other groups. These shared views have already contributed to the earlier sections.

1. Fathers

Some of the fathers interviewed felt that they weren't really fathers until their baby was born although they saw their partners as 'mothers already'. They generally felt they were just waiting and that there wasn't much they could do until after the birth. Some talked of the excitement of the scan:

> You felt a father then – you were on a bit of a high for a couple of days but after that I lapsed back.

In relation to their partners, some men felt they were being more considerate and helpful than usual:

> a bit more caring and watch out for her but I don't want to molly-coddle her – I don't want to wrap her up in cottonwool.

Some mentioned preparing financially and budgeting for the time when they would only have one salary. Some first-time fathers saw fatherhood as a challenge and an exciting opportunity.

Most of the men had found the books on pregnancy, birth and child development interesting – especially the development of the foetus. They had wanted to be more involved in the antenatal classes, but had been invited only to one or two sessions.

One father mentioned that he would like to understand more about the breathing instructions so he could support his wife in labour more confidently.

All intended to be present at the birth of their child. One father said he would gladly reverse roles with his wife and stay at home to look after the baby if it were financially possible and reflected that he would miss out on some early developments of his child through being at work. All wished paternity leave was longer and was a right. Some acknowledged that the baby was likely to make a greater change in their partner's life – especially if she decided to stay at home with the child and not return to work.

Anxieties were experienced about sleeplessness in the early months of being a father and the stress of coping with tiredness and work. They felt that unlike women there were few or no obvious places for men to discuss their feelings about becoming a father.

2. Asian women

A striking feature of the discussion group with the Asian women, was that their comments about pregnancy centred almost entirely around their contact with the health service. This had obviously been a source of difficulty and anxiety for them. At times, a less than adequate service had left them with unmet needs.

The women talked about the confusion of going to the clinic or being in hospital, when there was no link worker or interpreter available. They also lamented the lack of Asian health professionals and the inadequacies of White health professionals. As one said:

> They don't explain – like if you don't know English they won't explain to you – they just do what they have to do and that's that – you can go.

Another talked of being in hospital after the delivery:

> They never explain to you – you go for the blood pressure or something, you might find your baby gone, taken to the nursery for the night. With my first baby I was really in a panic wondering where it was. It would be easier if they explained.

Language difficulties had also meant that some of the women had not gone to antenatal classes:

> The antenatal classes – they don't get anyone explaining to you in your own language. Most of us miss out on the classes.

Several women mentioned that the food they had had in hospital had not been appropriate, and others had not been able to see a female doctor.

3. Second-time parents

Most of this group were finding their pregnancy more tiring than the first time round. They had fewer opportunities for rest with another child around, and felt that sometimes the health professionals did not adapt their advice to take account of the existing child. Visits to the clinic or hospital were more demanding because of taking a child with you, or needing to arrange for a baby-sitter. Long journey times and long waiting times were a particular deterrent when having to take a child too.

Overall, they felt more confident and more informed than during their first pregnancy. However, those who had had a difficult pregnancy or birth said they felt less confident. Everyone observed that they got much less attention, care and support from both family and health professionals. It was assumed they 'knew it all' and could cope. This extended to antenatal classes which they felt they had not been encouraged to attend.

Several women expressed the need to talk about how a new baby would affect their existing child, and how best to set about preparing for this.

4. Afro-Caribbean women

Although one fifth of the parents who took part in the research were Afro-Caribbean, there were no comments made during the discussions which related their experiences to their race. This may have been because the Afro-Caribbean women took part in racially mixed groups, or because no questions were asked directly about how their race influenced their experiences. Unfortunately, funding levels did not allow the running of a separate Afro-Caribbean group.

3.6 Summary of key issues of relevance to parent education

Pregnancy

- Lack of information and advice in early pregnancy, particularly about diet.
- Anxieties and worries in early pregnancy not addressed by health professionals.
- Concerns about self-image and body image during the whole of pregnancy, largely ignored by health professionals.
- Lack of opportunities for open-ended discussion and questions, both during care and at classes.
- Women need to be seen as having equal needs to those of the baby, and to be treated as a person rather than a vehicle for the baby.
- Conflicting advice is common and hard to deal with.
- Inability to imagine what it is like after the birth, but in retrospect wishing this had been addressed antenatally.
- Anxiety about tests and lack of information and explanations about the results and what they mean.
- An overall tendency for health professionals to ignore or skim over social, emotional and psychological aspects of pregnancy.
- Lack of access to adequate or appropriate services, information and support for Asian women.
- Second-time parents' needs largely ignored.
- Lack of opportunities for fathers to discuss issues and anxieties.

Being a parent

- Concerns about body shape and body image.
- Anxieties about feeding and the need for support with both bottle and breast-feeding.
- Need for time and opportunities to talk about what being a parent is like, the adjustments and feelings involved.
- Anxiety over conflicting advice.
- Desire for continuity of contact and care from professionals.
- A feeling that there is an undue focus on the baby, and the mother's health and feelings are largely ignored.
- A need expressed for contact with other mothers, for postnatal groups.
- Difficulties in detecting childhood illnesses and in dealing with GPs over illnesses.
- Second-time mothers' often wrongly assumed to know it all.

Section 4: Antenatal classes

4.1 The uptake of antenatal classes

Attendance rates

Various studies in the 1980s report both attendance and non-attendance rates at antenatal classes. The two most recent large studies involving random samples of women having live births in Sunderland and Bath, found non-attendance rates of 57% and 21%, respectively (Taylor, 1985; Milner, 1987). In Belfast, a smaller study of 379 women found a non-attendance rate of 78% (McKnight and Merrett, 1986). However, these figures included women who had no knowledge of the classes. This is highly significant in itself for if women do not know about a service they cannot choose whether or not to use it. It also means that the number of women who actively decide not to go to classes is lower than the overall non-attendance figures might at first suggest. Thus, from the figures given in the Sunderland report, it is possible to break down the non-attendance figures into 18% who did not know about classes and 39% who chose not to attend. Likewise, in the Belfast study where 46% of women did not receive an invitation to attend classes, the percentage of women choosing not to attend can be calculated as 32%.

When the studies are looked at for attendance rates, the picture becomes quite confusing, with widely differing definitions of attendance being used, and an almost total lack of information about the numbers and kinds of classes which were on offer. For example, the Bath study reports a 79% attendance rate, with attendance meaning going to a minimum of one out of a possible ten classes (Taylor, 1985). For health professionals running classes, this is not a useful definition of attendance – it includes women who may have gone to only one or two classes which, for whatever reasons, is a poor uptake level of service. Going to only one class is also unlikely to have much educational impact on a woman.

The three studies which did look at different levels of attendance found a low percentage of women attending most or all of the classes. In Belfast only 15% of women attended between 5 and 8 classes (McKnight and Merrett, 1986), while in Southend (Cox, 1985) 28% attended 5 or more classes, and in Sunderland only 16% of women attended all classes (Milner, 1990). Full attendance is perhaps too stringent a criterion by which to judge the success of a service. By virtue of many classes being offered late in pregnancy, some women will inevitably miss some classes because of their health or an early delivery (Perkins, 1979; Perfrement, 1982).

Who does or does not attend?

Given the variation in the definitions of attendance used in the studies reported, and whether they include all mothers or only first-time mothers, it is difficult to make valid comparisons between studies as to the characteristics of attenders and non-attenders. Table 3 summarizes some of the relevant findings for the main studies considered.

Overall, women who attend classes are more likely than non-attenders to have the characteristics listed in Table 4.

Table 3: Characteristics of women attending classes

- Middle-class or skilled working-class backgrounds (Perkins, 1979; Adams, 1982; Perfrement, 1982; Husband, 1983; Taylor, 1985; Milner, 1987)
- Aged 20 or over (Perkins, 1979; Cox, 1985)
- Married or in a stable relationship (Perfrement, 1982; Milner, 1987)
- Have average/above average educational attainment (Perfrement, 1982; Husband, 1983)
- First-time mothers (Perkins, 1979; Boyd and Sellers, 1982; Milner, 1990)
- Belong to the majority White racial group (Adams, 1982; Newham Parents Forum, 1988).

Table 4: Characteristics of women not attending classes

- From semi-skilled or unskilled working class backgrounds
- Below average educational attainment
- Aged 19 and under
- Single
- Belong to an ethnic minority group
- Already have at least one child

Unfortunately, all the above studies analyse only single variables, so it is not possible to identify which combination of characteristics would apply to either attenders or non-attenders. Only one study assesses the predictive nature of different characteristics, and found that attendance was most strongly predicted by educational attainment (Husband, 1983). This was a stronger predictor than social class.

Overall, this picture probably confirms what many practitioners suspect and often voice, as 'those who attend aren't the women who really need it' (Hyde, 1982), suggesting that antenatal classes are not reaching certain sections of the population.

Reasons for not attending classes

There appear to be three main reasons why women do not attend classes:

- They are not invited or do not know about them
- They do not perceive the need to attend nor do they see the classes as relevant
- They face practical difficulties in attending

Lack of information about classes

The success rate of health visitors and midwives in publicizing antenatal classes is quite variable. In the Belfast study 46% of the women were not invited (McKnight and Merrett, 1986), compared with 28% in the Midlands study (Perkins, 1979), 17% in the Bath study (Taylor, 1985), 16% in the Sunderland study (Milner, 1990), 39% in the Southend study (Cox, 1985) and 2% in the Glasgow study (McIntosh, 1988). Interestingly, only Perkins (1979) compared knowledge of classes between different groups of women and found that while 72% of the sample said they were offered classes, only 66% of women under 20 or over 30, and 50% of single/separated/divorced women or those whose husbands were unemployed, were offered classes. She suggests that either these women needed more of a 'sales pitch' so that they took in information about classes, or they were perceived as unlikely to attend or as more difficult to work with in a group, and so were not offered classes at all. Whichever of these reasons is correct, it suggests that health professionals may be unconsciously rationing a service to certain groups and then blaming those same groups for not using the service.

Perkins' study (1979) also found that a woman was most likely to be offered a class if she was to be a first-time mother, and least likely if she already had children. This was irrespective of whether or not the women with existing children had been to classes in a previous pregnancy.

In many health authorities, the usual practice is to inform women about antenatal classes, at the booking visit at the antenatal clinic. In some areas this is followed up by a written invitation or women are given a publicity leaflet showing the times and places of classes. Classes are also often publicized by posters in clinics, health centres and hospitals. Women may need to book a place in advance, either verbally through the clinic or in writing by returning a reply slip from a leaflet/invitation. For other classes, women choose where and when to go and simply turn up at the first class. All of these methods of invitation have advantages and disadvantages, and may inadvertently encourage or discourage certain women. Several authors have noted the importance of reinforcing verbal information, which can easily be forgotten, with written information about classes (Rees, 1982a, b; Milner, 1990), and of giving information about classes on more than one occasion. Whilst the booking visit seems a natural occasion to inform women of classes, if this is early in the pregnancy, the classes may seem a long way off and be forgotten. Milner (1990) points out that women at the booking visit may be in an unfamiliar situation which could be stressful; it involves tests and examinations and a lot of information is given on these occasions. This may mean the woman is overloaded and therefore may not take in some information.

No need for classes

In three studies, the most frequent reason given for not attending classes can be broadly classified as not seeing a need to attend. Thus, in the Belfast study 58% of the non-attending women said they were already familiar with pregnancy and so did not want to go to classes (McKnight and Merrett, 1986). In the Bath study 39% felt that classes were not likely to be helpful (Taylor, 1985), and in the Glasgow study 48% said classes would not be worthwhile (McIntosh, 1988).

For the Bath and Belfast studies, it could be argued that this finding is not unreasonable, since mothers who had already had a child were included. Neither study mentions whether there were special classes or refresher courses for multiparous women, which could be seen as more relevant than the full programme of antenatal classes. Perkins (1979) cautions against assuming that multiparous women do not attend because they may have been to classes in a previous pregnancy. She found that only 53% of women who had had previous live births had been to classes in a previous pregnancy.

Given the earlier findings that certain groups of women are less likely to attend than others, it could be assumed that it is these groups which specifically need convincing about the need for classes. However, none of the studies analyse which women give which reasons for not attending. This is a significant drawback to the research, since action to encourage attendance may need to be different for different groups of women. One study however, does give some interesting clues. The Glasgow study (McIntosh, 1988), which was restricted to first-time working-class mothers, found a 48% non-attendance rate. Of these women, almost half (48%) did not perceive the classes to be worth while. This is the highest figure found for this reason for non-attendance in all the literature reviewed here. It may indicate that working-class women are more likely to perceive classes as irrelevant than middle-class women. Interestingly, McIntosh notes that most of the women had formed this view of the classes from what family and friends had said.

In contrast, a study in Redbridge found that 40% of women not attending classes said the professionals had not given them the impression that it was important (Adams, 1982). This appeared to be strongly related to social class, with only 6% of Class I giving this reason, compared with 22% of Class IV and 38% of Class V.

Milner (1990) suggests that some women misunderstand what classes are for by assuming that only women who are unwell or had problems in previous pregnancies needed to attend. Our research also suggests that for working-class women, and particularly those who are single, going to classes is equated with not being able to cope (see Section 3.3).

Practical difficulties

Many recent studies highlight practical difficulties which stop women from going to classes. These difficulties include transport to classes, inconvenient times and locations, the need for childcare, and lack of time due to other commitments or work (Perkins, 1979; Cox, 1985; Taylor, 1985; McKnight and Merrett, 1986; McIntosh, 1988). These are all factors which those planning classes need to take into account. Some of the studies shed interesting light on aspects of these difficulties. Perkins (1979) found that the strongest predictor of non-attendance was having other children under the age of 5. At the same time, few of the classes had crèche provision or allowed young children in the classes, so that most women had to make special childcare arrangements in order to attend. Similarly, Curtice and Catley (1990) noted in a study in Liverpool that only one class offered a crèche and many of the community clinics where classes were held did not have play areas.

In Sunderland, attendance at classes was analysed for each of 15 health centres where women went to antenatal clinics. Interestingly two out of the four health centres which did not offer classes were in areas of disadvantage with many social problems. Non-attendance at classes was very high for people living in both these areas (73% and 78%), where women would have had to travel to get to classes at another health centre (overall non-attendance rates varied from 24% to 78%).

Reasons for stopping attending classes

Only three studies have looked at why women drop out of classes (Perkins, 1979; Hillier and Slade, 1989). For some women late booking into classes meant that they delivered before the end of the classes, whilst others gave birth early. In Perkins' study, of the 33% who dropped out, almost one third had given birth before completing the classes. Perkins also noted that some class teachers left particularly important topics, such as breast-feeding, to the end of the sequence of classes, so that they would be remembered better. However, the effect of this was to exclude a sizeable minority of women from learning about particularly important topics.

In a study in Sunderland, Milner (1990) found that absence rates for individual class sessions varied between 6% and 9%. The most common reason for absence was sickness, followed by family commitments. Absence rates were high (18%) for the first class, largely because some women were still working or found out about classes only after they had started.

Fathers and partners

Most of the literature focuses on the attendance patterns of women only. Four studies include brief information on fathers and partners attending classes. The levels of attendance at any classes are reported as low: 12% in the Redbridge study (Adams, 1982), 28% in Newham (Newham Parents Forum, 1988) and 36% in Bath (Taylor, 1985). In Perfrement's study (1982) 11% of partners had attended the full set of classes, and 32% had attended a fathers' evening only, leaving 68% who had no preparation through classes.

Take-up is clearly related to availability – in Redbridge 28% of classes were reported as not even having an evening for fathers, while in Bath two-thirds of the fathers had been offered only one or two sessions. Taylor notes a similar difference in the male take-up rate according to social class, as for the women in her study. Boyd and Sellers (1982) also found that 30% of women said their partners were not encouraged to attend.

As for the reasons for not attending, both Taylor and Adams found the most common to be that classes would not be helpful. Comments included a lack of interest and that attendance was not seen as part of a father's role. However, Taylor found that the belief that classes were not helpful was less common among fathers of first-time babies (25%, compared with 38% of all fathers) and suggests that this may indicate that fathers' attitudes are changing.

A significant obstacle to attending is the timing of classes during the day (Boyd and Sellers, 1982). Taylor (1985) found that 29% of non-attending fathers said the timing was inconvenient, and that this was mentioned most often by the working-class fathers.

Finally, the Southend study reports on women's views about fathers attending classes (Cox, 1985). A small minority of women (16%) felt it was very important for partners to come, which contrasted with 22% who thought it was not important at all. The main reasons why the fathers were thought not to attend were the inconvenient timing of classes and not being invited. Overall, 75% of class attenders felt that fathers were not encouraged to attend.

Parents from ethnic minority groups

Several studies report very low levels of attendance by women from ethnic minority groups. Adams (1982) found that only 1–6% of the different groups attended, whilst Jain (1985) reports a 2% attendance rate for Asian women, and

Firdous and Bhopal (1989) a 7% attendance rate for Asian women compared with 54% for a matched non-Asian control group. Newham Parents Forum (1988) report that only 20% of Asian women went to classes compared with an overall figure of 43%. Woollett and Dosanjh-Matwala (1990a, b) however, report that about half of a group of Asian women in the East End of London had attended a class for at least one of their pregnancies.

Both Jain (1985) and Woollett and Dosanjh-Matwala (1990a, b) note that those who spoke fluent English were the most likely Asian women to attend, and that often these were the younger women who had been educated in the United Kingdom. Lower attendance rates for Asian men were also found by Newham Parents Forum (1988): 15% attended compared with an overall rate of 28%.

The reasons given by Asian women for non-attendance include:

- Lack of knowledge about the classes or their likely benefit (Jain, 1985; Firdous and Bhopal, 1989)
- The need to look after children at home (Jain, 1985)
- Language barriers (Adams, 1982; Jain, 1985)
- A reluctance to go out at night, or difficulties in being accompanied to a day class (Newham Parents Forum, 1988).

Improving attendance at classes

Given the patterns of attendance at classes outlined in the previous section, it is clear that there is considerable room for improvement. At the most basic level, a significant minority of women do not get to know about the availability of classes. Suggestions to improve this situation include: having both verbal and written invitations to classes (Perkins, 1979; Rees, 1982a, b; Milner, 1990); telling women about classes on more than one occasion (Milner, 1990); making sure that health professionals do not offer classes selectively to particular groups of women, who are assumed to be the most interested or most likely to come (Perkins, 1979; Adams, 1982); targeting those least likely to come with information and reminders about classes in all the languages appropriate to the local area (Maternity Services Advisory Committee, 1984).

Even amongst women who do know about classes, there are again a substantial minority who elect not to attend for reasons of seeing no need/relevance or because of practical difficulties. Suggestions for tackling these obstacles include:

- More careful explanation to women as to what the classes are for, emphasizing their benefits and relevance (Adams, 1982; Maternity Services Advisory Committee, 1984; Taylor, 1985; McKnight and Merrett, 1986; Milner, 1990; McIntosh, 1988)
- More careful provision of targeted classes, particularly for multiparous women, fathers/partners and young mothers (Cox, 1985; Taylor, 1985)
- Offering classes in the evening as well as during the day to enable working parents and fathers to attend (Adams, 1982; Maternity Services Advisory Committee, 1982; Rees, 1982a, b; Husband, 1983; Cox, 1985; Taylor, 1985; McIntosh, 1988)

- Offering more local community classes so that less effort and expense is involved in getting to classes (Rees, 1982a, b; Husband, 1983; Jain, 1985; Milner, 1990; McIntosh, 1988)
- Provision of crèches or play areas, and welcoming children to classes to encourage women with children to attend (Perkins, 1979; Adams, 1982; Jain, 1985; Milner, 1987)
- Renaming classes to make them sound more attractive and relevant to parents (Dunwoody and Watters, 1990)
- Starting classes earlier in pregnancy to avoid non-completion due to early deliveries or late bookings (Perkins, 1979; Adams, 1982; Rees, 1982a, b)
- Providing classes or one-to-one education in hospital wards for those who have long stays in hospital before delivery (Maternity Services Advisory Committee, 1984)
- Targeting effort at particular groups seen as unlikely to attend without special encouragement (Rees, 1982; Milner, 1987)
- Targeting certain groups of women who are unlikely to attend, for home visits prior to classes (Husband, 1983)
- Recognizing the influence of family and friends on decisions about class attendance, and including them in conversations about classes, e.g. during home visits (McIntosh, 1988)
- See Section 7.2 for ideas relating to parents from ethnic minority groups.

A number of authors discuss the importance of setting antenatal classes into the wider context of the whole experience of antenatal care. The high number of routine visits that pregnant women are expected to make to clinics is widely discussed. Given that attendance at clinics is generally high some authors suggest that classes should be offered to coincide with clinics (McKnight and Merrett, 1986; Bishop, 1988; McIntosh, 1988). This should increase the likelihood of going to the classes as women are already there for the clinic, and would also decrease the overall effort, time and expense involved in going to classes and clinics as a whole.

Finally, it is important to note that whilst many suggestions have been made for ways to improve attendance at classes, there is little or no evaluation of the effectiveness of these ideas in practice. Anecdotal evidence abounds that certain strategies do help (for example, special groups targeted at young women – see Section 7.1). The only study to demonstrate a clear impact on antenatal class attendance was in Newcastle, as part of the Community Midwifery Care Project (Evans, 1991). This was a relatively long-term project aimed at providing an enhanced home-based community midwifery service to women living in two areas of social and economic deprivation. The impact on women involved in the project was compared with a control group of similar women in the same area. For those women in the project, the midwives had time to actively recruit for the classes, by reminding them verbally about classes whenever they saw them and putting reminder notes through their doors. The project found much higher attendance rates at classes among these women – 31% attending some classes, compared with only 4% of the control women. It also showed that the project had encouraged greater attendance for the project women, compared with their previous pregnancies when only 4% had attended classes. The evaluation also highlighted that the classes were more informal and the curriculum wider, focusing on the particular needs of the group, than previous classes, which may also have helped to increase attendance. These classes were also particularly successful in attracting teenage mothers, of whom 38% attended classes.

4.2 Parents' views about classes

Before reviewing the fairly large number of 'consumer' surveys of antenatal classes, it is important to remember that these provide only a partial view of what is being provided. McIntosh (1989) and other authors have pointed out that consumers tend to assume a service is well-founded and therefore the best that can be provided, and lack awareness of alternatives. This means that expressions of satisfaction are as often to do with low expectations as with positive feelings about the services.

The benefits

Four surveys have attempted to gauge women's general level of satisfaction with antenatal classes by asking them to rate the helpfulness of classes. Overall, between two-thirds and three-quarters of class attenders tend to rate classes as 'helpful' to 'very helpful' (Adams, 1982; Cox, 1985; Newham Parents Forum, 1988; Milner, 1990). This is not surprising, given that in these studies these were the comments of women who had continued to attend classes.

When asked which aspects of the classes were most helpful or best liked three themes emerge:

- Learning relaxation and breathing exercises
- Learning about pregnancy and labour
- Meeting other women

However, variations also exist between studies: for instance, Taylor (1985) found high ratings for learning about pregnancy and labour, whilst Adams (1982) noted that very few women valued any of the educational content of the classes compared with breathing/relaxation and meeting other women. Not surprisingly, Adams also found that 21% of the class attenders did not feel fully prepared for labour despite having attended classes.

In two studies which attempted to assess whether classes helped parents with the experiences of birth and early parenthood, the breathing and relaxation were seen by the large majority (85–87%) as having helped during labour (Cox, 1985; McIntosh, 1988). Taylor (1985) also found that the mothers who had attended classes rated the breathing/relaxation exercises as significantly more beneficial than mothers who had not been to classes.

A number of studies report that parents felt classes were good if they provided information and if they reduced worry or anxiety levels about labour (Perfrement, 1982; McIntosh, 1988; Newham Parents Forum, 1988).

The content of classes

There are a number of areas of criticism which the studies highlight to varying degrees.

- Lack of teaching about childcare
- Understanding about parenting is badly covered
- Unrealistic expectations not dispelled
- Lack of advice on how to avoid negative feelings and experiences
- Unrealistic preparation for labour
- Failure to recognize individual's circumstances

Lack of teaching about childcare

This is a common finding, with parents rating preparation for childcare poorly relative to labour and birth. Taylor (1985), for instance, found 25% of women felt that classes had been of little or no help on childcare, despite 51% finding them very or fairly helpful overall. Cox (1985), however, found that this did not apply to infant feeding, for which 90% of women thought the teaching was adequate or good. This contrasted with 65% of women thinking that there was not enough teaching on coping with a crying baby. Taylor (1985) noted that some parents were requesting instruction in practical skills such as feeding, bathing and changing nappies.

Understanding about parenting

This, again, is an area which parents feel classes do not cover well. The highest level of dissatisfaction in Taylor's study, was on understanding the parental role, for which 39% of women found classes to be of little/no help. Cox (1985) also found high percentages of women rating teaching on parenting as insufficient, even though only one third felt that classes had not helped in adjusting to motherhood. Dissatisfaction was highest for some of the social and emotional aspects of parenting – coping with a crying baby (65%), effect on income (63%), effects on social life (54%), moodiness (54%) and becoming a family (43%). Women in the research reported in Section 3.3 also wanted more time given to the postnatal period, and to the feelings and experiences of parents at this time.

Unrealistic expectations

Several studies report women as saying that the classes did nothing to dispel unrealistic expectations of parenting. Whilst some said the class content was itself unrealistic or lacking in practical detail (Newham Parents Forum, 1988; Perfrement, 1982), others said that an overall lack of teaching on parenting and childcare meant that existing unrealistic expectations remained intact (Taylor, 1985).

Avoiding negative feelings and experiences

Again a number of studies report that women criticize classes for avoiding or glossing over negative feelings and experiences in both pregnancy and after the birth (Newham Parents Forum, 1988). Perfrement (1982) notes that the postnatal period is rarely simple and problem-free, and quotes parents who felt guilty about their negative feelings because they had not realized this was a common experience. Women in our research (see Section 3.3) also said that difficult topics and anxieties tended to be avoided in classes, despite them wanting to discuss them.

Unrealistic preparation for labour

As reported earlier, many parents rate classes highly in helping to prepare for labour. However, few classes appear adequately to prepare women for the complications they may experience in labour, focusing instead on a straightforward and largely problem-free labour (Perfrement, 1982; Taylor, 1985; Newham Parents Forum, 1988). Several studies report that it is largely the parents who experience these complications who complain about the classes omitting to cover them (Draper *et al.*, 1982; Perfrement, 1982; Taylor, 1985).

Some studies also report that classes do not prepare women adequately for the pain levels involved in childbirth (Cartwright, 1985; Taylor 1985), but may mislead some women into thinking that, if the breathing and relaxation exercises are used, labour will be relatively pain-free.

Several studies also comment that the classes do not always prepare women for the realities of being in hospital (Gillet, 1985) or that the procedures experienced were different from what they had been led to believe from the classes (Cartwright, 1985).

Failure to recognize circumstances of individuals

Several studies report criticism from some parents that classes do not take on board the variety in parents' circumstances. Evans (1991) notes that some women did not go to classes because the information and advice was not geared to their low income levels.

Information needs

Several studies report differing views on how far classes meet women's needs for information. Whilst the majority of women appear to find classes very informative, there may be a minority who find the information too simple or at the wrong level (Perfrement, 1982; Milner, 1990; Newham Parents Forum,

1988). Some studies also report parents as saying that teaching needs to be more down to earth and practical (Taylor, 1985). One study notes that some parents find classes organized by the National Childbirth Trust (NCT) more informative and able to cover topics more in-depth than health service classes (Boyd and Sellers, 1982).

A study by Ball (1989) suggests that classes are felt to be most helpful in terms of meeting information needs by working-class women and those in council housing – in fact, those groups generally least likely to attend classes.

Teaching methods and ethos of classes

Parents' views about the teaching methods and ethos of classes have been investigated much less than their views about the content and topics covered. Several studies report parents as valuing time for discussion and opportunities to ask questions (Perfrement, 1982; Cox, 1985; Taylor, 1985). These same studies note that in some classes discussion was felt by parents to be unsuccessful because of a number of factors: the group size was too big; the group changed from week to week; and the setting or the group leader did little to put people at ease. Boyd and Sellers (1982) also found that parents valued, but rarely had opportunities for, in-depth discussion in health service classes, but that this was more usual in NCT classes.

Parents' comments on the use of audio-visual aids, suggest that sometimes they are not integrated into class teaching (Cox, 1985), that they may be out of date or paint too rosy a picture of birth or children (Perfrement, 1982; Taylor, 1985) and that parents value the discussion provoked by a film as much if not more than the film itself (Perfrement, 1982).

The approach of the class leader is commented on by parents in several studies. Some parents in Taylor's study felt that their class leaders lacked good teaching skills and that they were not always able to provide practical and down to earth information. Suggestions for improvements include the need for class leaders to have had children themselves (Taylor, 1985; Newham Parents Forum, 1988).

Some parents also clearly value time to chat to other parents informally, and share experiences and stories (Boyd and Sellers, 1982). For some parents, this appears to be as useful or more so than the more formal parts of a session (Perfrement, 1982).

Fathers and partners

Whilst the majority of studies have been of women's views of antenatal classes, two do report on fathers' views. Taylor (1985) found that, for the minority of fathers who attended classes, teaching about birth and relaxation exercises was rated most highly, although not as highly as by the mothers. Some fathers commented that there was not enough on how fathers can help women in labour and with their breathing, a finding mirrored in the Newham study (Newham Parents Forum, 1988). Around half the fathers in Taylor's study had found classes to be of very little or no help on childcare or the parental role. This probably reflects the fact that fathers were generally offered only one or two sessions, which tended to focus on labour and birth. Some fathers also felt marginalized or patronized in classes, and commented that their role was often ignored or underplayed by the class leaders.

It is also interesting to note studies that report anecdotal evidence from women that they feel benefits from fathers going to classes. Butler (1985) reports that on asking mothers postnatally about classes, they valued fathers attending because it increased the likelihood of them attending the birth or of being supportive during labour. Conversely, Perfrement (1982) reports that some women felt their partners did not cope well with being at the birth, because they had not gone to classes and did not know what to expect.

Parents from ethnic minority groups

Only two studies report feedback from women of ethnic minority groups on what they felt about antenatal classes. This may be because so few women from ethnic minority groups actually attend classes (see Section 4.1). Woollett and Dosanjh-Matwala (1990a, b) found that most Asian women who went to classes felt they were useful, and particularly the first-time mothers. Most saw classes as primarily educational, but several women felt they had a more social and support function. Most of the women from four different Asian groups in Jain's study (1985) did not go to classes, but did suggest ways of making them more accessible:

- Hold classes locally within walking distance
- Have an Asian leader, who spoke appropriate languages and was trained in parent education
- Have playworkers to look after other children

The women also suggested a greater role for their GPs in parent education, since most of the GPs were Asian.

The timing of classes in pregnancy

A significant minority of parents express the wish to have classes starting earlier on in pregnancy. Cox (1985) found that 27% of class attenders would have liked to have gone earlier, while Perfrement (1982) notes an expressed need for classes at 4–5 months for some women. The fact that a minority of women do not complete courses for reasons of giving birth or going into hospital because of complications (Perkins, 1979; Perfrement, 1982) also suggests that earlier classes might suit some women. However, studies also report that women want classes to start once they leave work (Perfrement, 1982), which could militate against the take up of classes offered earlier in pregnancy.

Variations in parents' views

Unfortunately there is very little in the literature to indicate how different groups of parents vary in their expressed views of classes. Taylor (1985), however, did find that working-class parents were generally more appreciative of classes than middle-class parents. This was particularly noticeable in how they rated teaching about childcare – this was rated as fairly/very helpful by over half the working-class parents compared to only one fifth of the middle-class parents. Studies otherwise report parents' views *en bloc* without analysing them according to variables which may be significant, such as age, marital status and ethnic group.

Improvements to classes

The following list summarizes ways in which parents feel classes could be improved, and includes improvements suggested by professionals on the basis of parents' views about the classes:

- More emphasis on childcare and living with a new baby (Adams 1982; Cox, 1985; Taylor, 1985), including teaching care skills (Taylor, 1985).
- More emphasis on the role of a parent, including social and psychological adjustments (Adams, 1982; Cox, 1985; Taylor, 1985).
- Acknowledging negative as well as positive feelings and experiences, both in pregnancy and after the birth (Adams, 1982).
- Using the experiences of a newly delivered mother to help women increase their understanding of the postnatal period (Draper *et al.*, 1982; Perfrement, 1982; Cox, 1985; Taylor, 1985).
- More information about labour complications and what can go wrong (Cox, 1985; Perfrement, 1984).
- Promoting realistic expectations of labour pain levels (Cartwright, 1985) and of the postnatal period (Draper *et al.*, 1982).
- More emphasis on the role of partners in labour (Taylor, 1985) and of the father's role during pregnancy and after the birth (Cox, 1985; Taylor, 1985).
- An equal emphasis given to the needs and experiences of the parent and the baby (see Section 3.3).
- A greater emphasis on the social, emotional and psychological aspects of pregnancy and parenting (see Section 3.3).

4.3 Professionals' views about antenatal classes

The literature on professionals' views about classes is limited to only a handful of studies. Extensive use is therefore made of the issues raised by the interviews with professionals carried out for this review. Where appropriate, reference is also made to relevant issues raised incidentally in the rest of the literature on antenatal classes.

Dissatisfaction with classes

Two studies report that significant numbers of health visitors and midwives are dissatisfied with their own involvement in antenatal classes. McCabe *et al.* (1984) found that two-thirds of midwives and one third of health visitors were dissatisfied with classes. Rees (1982a, b), in a survey of 39 health visitors and midwives, found that 67% were dissatisfied with some aspect of classes. A number of linked issues appear to account for this dissatisfaction. These are detailed in the rest of this section.

Identifying and meeting needs

More flexible provision needed

Overall, the professionals interviewed were very aware that antenatal classes are not generally taken up by the majority of pregnant women. They stressed the need for more flexible provision, emphasizing particularly the need for:

- Classes at different locations and times, and particularly in the evenings, to accommodate working parents.
- Classes designed to meet the special needs of certain groups, such as young women and women whose first language is not English.

There was a general recognition that in many areas classes are geared to and taken up by largely middle-class, educated White women. This generated a concern that 'those who need it most don't come' or that 'we only get the converted'. Similar sentiments are reported in much of the literature (for example, Rees 1982; McCabe *et al.*, 1984).

Too many needs

Many professionals felt it was easy to identify a long list of topics and issues which need to be covered, particularly if classes are to prepare women adequately for their experiences of pregnancy, birth and parenting. Several expressed feelings of frustration that there were so many needs, which it was impossible to cover in six or eight classes. They felt it was important for this to be acknowledged, so that antenatal classes were not set up to fail by being seen as the answer to all educational needs.

Whose agenda?

A strong and recurring theme in the interviews was that health professionals wanted to work to the agendas of pregnant women. This is also reflected in some of the literature (for example, Billingham, 1989; Clements, 1989). This was seen as an important part of 'consumer satisfaction' and one significant reason why in the past, women may have been put off coming to classes with a set format. However, there was an ambivalence about how far the agendas of women should influence the content of classes. An entirely women-led agenda was seen by most as not desirable. They felt that pregnant women do not always know their own needs, and that part of the health professional's role is to contribute what they knew from past experience women would find useful. A commonly cited example related to postnatal experiences. The professionals repeatedly observed that women find it very hard to think about the period after the birth – this was summed up as the 'brick wall of labour'. A women-led agenda would therefore be unlikely to raise this issue. However, in retrospect women often wished that classes had tackled this topic. Health professionals also felt that they had a legitimate professional agenda, based on the priorities of the health service to which they needed to work and for which they were accountable.

Fears were also expressed that, if agendas were negotiated, health professionals taking classes might not have the expertise or knowledge to respond to some of the women's requests. Alternatively, women might ask to spend time on something felt to be relatively unimportant. Given that most people felt there was never really enough time to cover even the basics, this was a significant fear.

Meeting individual needs

Several people felt that classes were poor at meeting individual needs. The general approach was to focus on common needs and so 'teach to the middle'. However, this meant that some women had unmet needs. One solution to this was seen as using a more participative approach: if a group was encouraged to contribute their views and experiences as an integral part of a session, they would influence how any topic was addressed, and be more likely to meet their own needs.

The 'because it's there' syndrome

A general resistance to change was identified by a number of people as an obstacle to thinking about how well classes meet women's needs. There was an attitude that 'we've always done it this way and no one's ever complained', or that women turning up to classes was proof that everything was all right as it was. In addition several people felt there was sometimes a tendency to add topics to classes, not on the basis of need, but because there was someone locally who could come and 'do a good session' on a particular topic.

The content of classes

Over-emphasis on information

The majority of the professionals interviewed felt that classes were geared too much to giving information to pregnant women. Whilst some information was essential, it was felt that there were quicker and more effective ways of providing some of this information – for example, through using handouts or having videos available for people to borrow and use at home. This would then free up some time for considering other issues, such as the emotional aspects of becoming a parent, which are more appropriately considered in a group setting.

Several people also noted that some health professionals have a tendency either to present partial information and advise on certain courses of action, or simply to present all the information in a neutral manner. What was needed by women was the information plus an opportunity to think through various choices or courses of action and their consequences. Partial information or the full information was not of itself felt to be particularly useful. This is also emphasized by Clements (1989), who notes that women already bring much knowledge with them to classes, and so do not need to receive a body of knowledge. Instead they need help to satisfy their own individual needs in relation to this body of knowledge.

'Keeping it light' versus tackling the negatives

There was a clear dichotomy among those interviewed on this issue. Some felt strongly that the overall effect of classes must be to reassure women and that this is achieved only by stressing the positive aspects of pregnancy and the early months of parenthood. It was therefore important to play down difficulties and counter negative attitudes or experiences. In contrast, others felt equally strongly that this approach does not prepare women for the realities ahead, and that it is better to acknowledge and discuss openly difficulties and negative experiences, as well as more positive ones. If women have been alerted to these possibilities in advance – for example, having angry feelings towards the baby – they are less likely to feel guilty about difficult experiences and more likely to cope constructively. Some of the more uncomfortable or negative experiences mentioned were miscarriage, stillbirth, complicated labour, handicap, postnatal depression and sexuality.

Emotional and social aspects

Most of those interviewed felt that classes generally spent insufficient time on the emotional and social aspects of pregnancy, birth and parenting. Reasons for this varied, and included a lack of confidence, a lack of training, feeling less comfortable with these aspects than with a straight information role and feeling powerless because there were no clear solutions or answers to be offered.

These views are also echoed in the literature (Redbridge and Waltham Forest Area Health Education Service, 1980; Clements, 1989). Holden (1990) suggests that better coverage of emotional aspects of becoming a parent with both men and women could help to improve postnatal experiences.

Inappropriate timing

A number of people felt that classes should not cover nutrition, smoking, alcohol and drug use, because they were run too late in pregnancy for women to make changes which might affect their baby's health. Others, however, felt it was still worth doing so in the hope of influencing the woman's health beyond pregnancy, and particularly in a future pregnancy.

Several articles also recommend that babycare should be taught postnatally rather than antenatally, so as to coincide with the time of need (Perkins, 1979; Adams, 1982).

Teaching methods and resources

A range of methods

Most people saw the need to balance three main teaching methods:

- Information giving – usually done by a talk from a health professional, often quite informally, or by showing a video.
- Group discussion – often following or integrated with giving information.
- Practical – parents practising practical skills, usually of breathing and relaxation, but also sometimes childcare skills.

In talking about teaching methods, discussion was mentioned most often as the method which people find difficult. Problems included large group size or room size and layout mitigating against discussion; difficulties in getting some groups or some women to participate; a lack of time; getting off the point; and worrying about how to counter misinformation or negative experiences contributed by parents in discussion.

Rees (1982a, b) also found, from a questionnaire with health visitors and midwives, that lack of teaching skills were found to be the most difficult aspect of running classes for most people. Difficulties included handling discussion, matching information to individual needs and coping with individuals' anxieties constructively. Interestingly, a study of interactions within classes found that some teachers were very quick to fill silences or pauses, and did not give women enough time to think before speaking – 29% of class teachers paused for less than 3 seconds after asking a question before carrying on talking (Murphy-Black, 1986).

Several of those interviewed also talked about using structured group work activities, in which small groups undertook a task which was discussed and de-briefed by the whole group. This kind of approach was seen as enabling women to learn from one another as much as from a health professional, as well as gaining confidence in themselves and support from one another. There was, however, felt to be a significant lack of published material to support this approach and a lack of training in the running of participatory group work.

Some of those interviewed also expressed concern about whether to invite a new mother to talk to the group about the experiences of birth and the early months of motherhood. Whilst people knew that parents found this valuable, they also worried about what might be said, with the implication that parents might learn the 'wrong things'.

A similar point about how to make the best use of individual experiences was raised in relation to the experiences of the individual health professional taking the class. The dilemma was that parents often wanted to know what the class leader had herself experienced, whilst the class leaders felt they should be trying to put across a range of views and experiences. Giving undue emphasis to the personal experience of the leader was seen as poor practice, but also an area which people often found hard to deal with appropriately.

Social contact

Strictly speaking, the social contact fostered between women during classes is not a teaching method. However, a number of those interviewed felt that women gain a lot from the informal contact with other women, during coffee breaks, and at the start and finish of sessions. Several people felt this contact was as important a time for learning, through the sharing of experiences and views with people in a similar situation, as the more formal part of the session. They felt classes should be structured to foster this contact, through long breaks or by using activities which women could do in small groups. Other small ways of fostering social support were also felt to be often missed – for instance encouraging women to exchange addresses or telephone numbers.

Parents' expectations

This was mentioned frequently as an obstacle to using participative teaching methods. Many people had observed that parents come to classes expecting talks in which they are largely passive receivers of information. These expectations were seen as arising largely from experiences of school. Interestingly, this was also given as a significant reason for why some women choose not to come to classes – those who had disliked school or not achieved at school being the ones most likely to be put off by an expectation that classes would be like school.

Appropriate resources

Overall there was felt to be a lack of appropriate resources to support parent education. For some people, this was because of budgetary restrictions, which meant that resources which existed could not be used – for example, handouts of information. Others felt that the resources they needed did not exist. This was mentioned largely in relation to resources which were relevant to the very wide range of social, economic, cultural and family backgrounds of pregnant women today. Current resources were still felt to be geared to nuclear families and to offer little help to the practitioner on how to set information about pregnancy and parenting into the appropriate and varying contexts of parents' lives.

A particularly significant resource which was lacking for practitioners working in certain areas was access to an interpreter. This was mentioned as the main reason for not being able to run classes for parents whose first language was not English. McCabe *et al.* (1984) also report practitioners' lack of access to interpreters as a key reason for not providing classes especially for Asian women.

Finally, there were quite a number of comments about the appropriate use of video. Views varied as to how far video should be used, but it was a common perception that parents expected and liked to see videos. There were, however, considerable difficulties in some areas, in being able to get hold of videos, due to competition between health professionals for the same resources. This led in some places, to videos needing to be booked six or more months in advance. This in turn meant that the programme for the classes became fixed and lacked the flexibility to either respond to group requests or to re-order sessions based on group needs. There was a strong impression that in some areas, the organization and structure of antenatal classes had become dominated to a significant degree by the need to ensure access to scarce video resources. Similar problems with access to and use of up-to-date audio-visual material are also reported in the literature (Rees, 1982a, b).

Unclear aims

In a survey of 50 health visitors and midwives involved in antenatal education in Redbridge and Waltham Forest (1980), a very large majority (98%) were found not to have clear or achievable aims for their teaching. Aims were also found to vary amongst staff and were all concerned with what health professionals hoped to achieve rather than with what parents might get out of classes.

Changing groups

Several people mentioned that when classes are organized on a continuous basis, with parents joining and leaving as they choose, the fostering of a supportive group climate becomes difficult. Fixed groups with a definite start and finish with a set group of women were preferred and felt to be more educationally effective. However, as the Redbridge study also notes (1980) fixed groups are sometimes hard to arrange, without some women missing out on beginning classes at an appropriate stage in their pregnancy.

Large numbers were also felt to be counter-productive educationally, but people knew that groups upwards of 20 or 30 people are still quite common.

Organization and management

Obstacles to flexible provision

Despite an awareness of the need to provide classes at a range of times and locations there appeared to be a number of significant obstacles to this happening. The two most important issues related to classes run in the evening: staff found it hard and sometimes impossible to get time off in lieu for evening work; and it was difficult to get safe access to premises, and particularly community health service premises in the evening.

Some people also noted an unwillingness amongst colleagues and managers to try out new ways of offering classes. The most common reason given for this was past experience, that 'we try and offer them what they [parents] say they want and then they don't turn up'. Staff often seemed to be under-estimating the amount of time and effort which is needed in planning and publicizing something new, and seemed to hold on to a belief that if a service is provided it should and will be used by parents.

This suggested an underlying problem of staff attitudes to women who do not take up antenatal classes. It was felt that commonly women were blamed for not coming to classes usually because they did not see them as relevant, interesting or desirable. The practical difficulties which some women face in attending classes were felt to be underplayed, and therefore rarely influenced how classes were planned and organized locally.

The survey by McCabe *et al.* (1984) also found practical obstacles to flexible provision – unsuitable venues and accommodation and numbers attending not matching the space available. However, they found that practitioners were well aware of the practical obstacles preventing women from attending classes. There was some degree of frustration expressed that organizational problems prevented more flexible provision which could help to attract women who had difficulties in attending.

Staffing

A number of staffing issues were raised in the interviews, issues which caused frustration and were seen as hindering good work practice. The most important of these was how work rotas for health visitors and midwives are organized. In some areas rotas seem to mitigate against the same individual being able to lead a particular class from beginning to end. It was also reported that crises or poor planning meant that staff were not infrequently diverted to other work, with a colleague being asked to stand in at short notice. This makes continuity within a class difficult. The need for colleagues to be able to stand in for one another at short notice had contributed in some areas to a decision to standardize classes to a set format and order.

Rees (1982a, b) also found that involvement in classes was often on a rota basis, so that an individual practitioner took a class only once every 12–18 months. This lack of continuity meant that practitioners felt they could not easily build on and use their experience of running one set of classes to improve future classes.

Although rivalry between health visitors and midwives in parent education is apocryphal, and does feature in the literature (for example, Rees 1982a, b), the professionals interviewed felt that this had been much reduced in recent years. Despite obvious variations in how far health visitors and midwives work together, it was generally felt that both had an important role to play, and both contributed equally valid skills and perspectives. Midwives were often seen as having expert knowledge of birth and hospital practices, whilst health visitors had particular expertise in health education and postnatal issues, and brought a useful understanding of each individual's circumstances and needs based on their experiences of working in local communities.

Budgets

These were reported as a significant difficulty in some areas. Budgets were either insufficient to allow the use of up-to-date resources or the provision of refreshments, or they were allocated inappropriately so that health visitors and midwives competed or had unequal access to resources. Limited budgets were also felt to be a major obstacle to starting new kinds of classes, or to experimenting with provision which was not guaranteed to show immediate results. The desire to have smaller group sizes to enable more participation and discussion meant running more classes which was impossible because of budgetary restrictions.

In the literature, Rees (1982a, b) reports on difficulties faced by practitioners in improving practice, following an intensive in-service training course. A lack of resources was found to be the most common block – resources of time, money and staff.

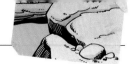

Staff training and support

The most frequently mentioned organizational issue which restricted the development of local practice, was a marked lack of opportunities for staff training and support. Many antenatal teachers had learnt 'on the job', having little or no initial or in-service training for this area of work. This was felt to be particularly important in the area of learning group work skills, which was reinforced by earlier comments about practitioners lacking skills and confidence for group discussion. A lack of appropriate training is also highlighted by Clements (1989) and by the Redbridge and Waltham Forest (1980) study, where 50% of practitioners felt their training to be inadequate for the job. McCabe *et al.* (1984) also found that 59% of midwives and 82% of health visitors expressed the wish for more training.

Of equal importance is a lack of time for practitioners to plan and prepare antenatal classes and to keep themselves up-to-date with local practices and ideas and information on health education, as noted also by Rees (1982a, b).

Practitioners were also felt to be often lacking support from either managers or colleagues. Managers commonly appeared to give low priority to antenatal education and therefore underestimated staff needs for support and training. People reported that it was often difficult for practitioners to get time for attending meetings, support groups or working parties. Practitioners, in turn, felt isolated and unsupported, a situation which was sometimes exacerbated by the negative attitudes of colleagues who saw classes as a 'soft option' and not the 'real work' of a health visitor or midwife.

One area where adequate time for liaison and updating is essential, is in community staff keeping themselves up-to-date with hospital procedures, so that classes properly reflect local practices (Redbridge and Waltham Forest Area Health Education Service, 1980).

Evaluation

A number of those interviewed felt that evaluation of antenatal education was an increasingly significant issue. Some noted that a lack of clarity about the aims of antenatal education was reflected in confusion about how best to approach its evaluation. There were also pressures in some areas to measure its success in terms of birth outcomes, reduced low birth weight or perinatal mortality rates, or in terms of changes in behaviour such as pregnancy smoking rates. Although some people felt these pressures may need resisting, there were relatively few ideas about what were appropriate outcome measures and how these might relate to the setting of targets and the drawing up of purchaser-provider contracts.

Whilst parent or 'consumer' satisfaction was seen as an important part of evaluation, there were some concerns about how exactly to do this and how much weight should be given to parents' views.

4.4 Special classes

Preconception, education and counselling

This involves advice for women who may be planning a pregnancy, about the kind of lifestyle which is thought to maximize the health of both mother and foetus (Staines, 1983). Although some areas reportedly offer preconception clinics (Williams and Booth, 1985; Gillies and Chaudhry, 1984), much of this area of work is probably covered in an informal way through the general work of health visitors, particularly with women who have already had a child.

Given that a significant minority of women do not become pregnant intentionally, the potential for preconception education is somewhat limited. A recent study in Belfast, for example, found that almost half of the women had not planned their pregnancy. Considerably more women who fell into an 'at risk' category based on socio-economic factors, had not planned their pregnancy compared with a 'not at risk' group (52% versus 32%) (McKnight and Merrett, 1986). This supports the reported notion (see, for example, Williams and Booth, 1985) that those groups which are 'at risk' and therefore could benefit from preconception education are those least likely to take it up since their pregnancies are more often unplanned.

Whilst some professionals appear to value the aims of preconception education, it does not seem to have great appeal to parents – from the professionals interviewed, it appears not to be a service currently in great demand by parents. McCabe *et al.* (1984) also noted that health professionals particularly doubted its relevance to working-class women. They also found a disparity in views about what focus it should take, ranging from a medical-behavioural focus to a social-psychological focus.

Early pregnancy classes

A one-off class may be offered to women early in their pregnancy, with its focus as the first trimester of pregnancy. For example, the West London Hospital offers a class to women between 8 and 20 weeks' pregnant, and covers the development of the baby, food and exercise for health, changes in lifestyle, benefits and the purpose of antenatal care (Gillet, 1985). In some areas the National Childbirth Trust also offers a similar class in recognition of the importance of the changes and decisions that occur in early pregnancy, when many women may not yet have started regular antenatal care (Precey, 1986). Whilst one early pregnancy session appears to be the norm in Britain, a recent survey of US childbirth educators reported a recommended length of four 2-hour sessions in order to cover the issues of concern to parents (Maybruck, 1988). However, the survey also noted difficulties of poor attendance. Ciliska

(1983) reports from Canada on a local early pregnancy class (three sessions of 1½ hours) which has a particular emphasis on enabling parents to assess their lifestyles and to identify and implement changes in relation to diet, smoking and exercise.

Aquanatal classes

A fairly recent innovation has been the introduction of aquanatal classes for women who are pregnant or have recently had a baby. Specially designed exercises are performed by women standing upright in shoulder-depth water. Aquanatal aims to help maintain and improve fitness, flexibility and muscle strength with a minimum of stress and to help reduce common complaints in pregnancy such as backache.

4.5 Recent innovations

In response to some of the dissatisfactions expressed by both parents and professionals about antenatal classes, a number of health authorities and individual practitioners have been involved in various initiatives designed to improve take-up rates and the quality of local classes.

Increasing choices

Some health authorities have aimed to increase the choice of times and locations at which classes are available, with increasing numbers offering classes in the evening to accommodate working parents.

Targeting

Poor attendance by certain groups of women have led to special classes being set up, in which the content and approach is adapted to meet particular needs. Common examples are classes for young women (see Section 7.1) or second-time parents (see Section 7.4).

A community midwifery project in Newcastle (Evans, 1991) also reports setting up classes for women from a similar socio-economic background, which enabled education to be focused on particular needs.

Better publicity and active recruitment

Survey findings indicating that some parents do not get invited to classes or do not perceive them as relevant, have led to health authorities reviewing their systems of publicity and invitation. Initiatives have included:

- Changing the title of classes, to avoid using words such as 'parentcraft' or 'classes' which may have technical or medical connotations, and using more ordinary language such as 'ready for baby' groups (Rees, 1982a, b).
- Producing attractive written information about classes to reinforce a verbal invitation, and to outline the purpose, content and benefits of attending classes (Rees, 1982,a b).
- Actively recruiting women to classes and reminding them as often as possible – in one special community midwifery project, midwives also put reminder notes through women's doors (Evans, 1991).

Widening the scope

In some areas the scope of classes has been widened in the hope of attracting women who are otherwise unlikely to attend. This has included:

- Providing practical activities such as cooking or swimming as part of a programme of classes (Evans, 1991).
- Providing for particular needs as requested by parents – for example, welfare and benefits advice (Billingham, 1989).
- Parents themselves preparing for and leading group discussions (Billingham, 1989).

Participative and informal style

A recognition that classes need to cover feelings, attitudes and skills as well as information has led to increased use of participatory teaching methods including discussion and structured small group work (for example, Clements, 1989).

Integrated care and education

In response to observations that the take-up rates for antenatal care are high compared with classes, some clinics now offer integrated care and education. Classes are timed to coincide with the start or finish of clinic sessions, so that women do not have to make extra effort to attend classes (Husband, 1983; McKnight and Merrett, 1986; Billingham, 1989).

Standardization

Various reports have recommended that antenatal classes become standardized across a health district, with a set length, order of topics and content (Cox, 1985;

Milner, 1987). This move to standardization has been in response to difficulties experienced by staff (such as lack of planning and preparation time, needing to deputize for one another at short notice) and comments from parents about variability in the content and quality of classes.

In-service training

A number of reports have identified the use of group work and communication skills as a priority for training for practitioners (Clements, 1989). The provision of such training is documented in several reports (Rees, 1982a, b; Murphy-Black and Faulkner, 1988).

Local working parties and support groups

Working parties or formal committees have been set up by some health authorities in order to review provision and identify priorities for change (for example, Clements, 1989). In other areas, practitioner support groups provide a forum for health professionals to get together to update themselves and support one another in developing their practice (for example, as reported for Halton Health Authority, in the professional interviews for this review).

Section 5: Education within antenatal care

Whilst a considerable amount of research has been devoted to assessing the effectiveness of antenatal classes, relatively little has been written about the educational opportunities provided within the system of antenatal care. The first report of the Maternity Services Advisory Committee (1982) identifies a number of general and specific educational needs, which antenatal care should aim to meet for all pregnant women in addition to 'parentcraft classes':

> Antenatal care should provide support and guidance at the time, and help them to prepare for parenthood (P.1)
>
> It is important for them to receive early advice on health matters such as diet, smoking, alcohol or drugs (P.4)
>
> All women need advice on how to respond to changes which they may notice and in particular what to do if various symptoms develop. They also need full information about how to recognise the onset of labour and what to do when that happens (P.11)
>
> It is generally agreed that breastfeeding should be discussed early in pregnancy and frequently thereafter (P.17)
>
> It is important that the reasons for procedures and tests, and their results and meaning, should be explained (P.17)
>
> All women need a service which treats their questions sympathetically (P.1)

The opportunities for health education are much less clearly defined within antenatal care than within antenatal classes. However, the take-up of antenatal care has repeatedly been reported as being very high, with a very large majority of women attending most, or all of their clinic appointments. This contrasts with the relatively low take-up rates reported for antenatal classes (see Section 4.1). It means that for a significant proportion of women (well over half in many areas) antenatal care provides the main opportunity for the health service to respond to and meet educational needs.

This acquires greater significance in the light of research which suggests that this group of women are likely to have less existing knowledge about pregnancy and birth (see Section 8.2), and are more likely to be from working-class or disadvantaged backgrounds (see Section 4.1) which itself tends to militate against full use of health services (Townsend and Davidson, 1982). Some authors also argue that it is also this group of women, who are at greater risk of obstetric and perinatal complications, who tend to have less healthy lifestyles and so are in fact in greater need of health education during pregnancy.

The remainder of this section attempts to evaluate how successful antenatal care has been in meeting the educational needs of women, from the viewpoints of both parents and professionals. Opportunities for health education theoretically exist on all occasions of antenatal care. Of particular significance and importance are the occasions when pregnancy is confirmed and the antenatal clinic booking visit.

5.1 The confirmation of pregnancy

Many women confirm their pregnancy with their general practitioner (GP) (or less often at a family planning clinic or well woman clinic), who is in an ideal position to provide information and advice about the early stages of pregnancy. At this stage an individual's pattern of drinking, smoking, drug use and diet are thought to be particularly influential on the healthy development of the foetus. Since women are not usually expected to attend the antenatal clinic until they are pregnant for 10–12 weeks or more, the GP will be the main or only health service contact in the early months of pregnancy. Moreover, there are consistent reports of a minority of women attending late for the antenatal clinic due to delays in GP referral – Perfrement (1982), for instance, reports that 20% of women in her study did not attend the antenatal clinic until they were more than 16 weeks pregnant. For these women the GP may have a particularly important educational role to play.

Despite the importance of the confirmation visit, there is relatively little research on how far GPs use this visit for health education. One recent study does suggest that many GPs do not use this visit to maximum effect (McCabe *et al.*, 1984). It found that the majority of GPs did not spend long enough on the confirmation visit for health education to be considered in much depth (14% spent less than 10 minutes; 75% spent 10–20 minutes; 7% spent more than 20 minutes). Moreover, many tended to concentrate on medical topics such as weight, smoking and rubella, to the exclusion of the emotional and social aspects of pregnancy. They were also found to take a rather negative and didactic approach to the advice they gave.

Specific evidence on what information and advice is offered to women by their GPs comes from Perfrement (1982), who found that only 20% received written and/or verbal advice about diet. In another large survey of pregnant women and smoking, only 40% had been given information about smoking or advice on how to give up by their GP (Madeley *et al.*, 1989). Advice about alcohol intake seems even rarer, with McKnight and Merrett (1987a) finding that only 4% of women had discussed their drinking with their GP. In this same study only 4% of women had had dietary advice from their GP, despite the fact that one third of them were found to have a nutritionally unbalanced diet during pregnancy (McKnight and Merrett, 1987b).

The wider role of GPs

Women may visit their GP at various times during pregnancy, all of which present opportunities for antenatal education. However, the Redbridge and Waltham Forest study (1980) found that despite two-thirds of women regularly visiting their GP during pregnancy, 60% of these women were not given advice by their GP, and only 32% found the advice they were given to be useful.

5.2 The booking visit

Slightly more research has considered the potential of the antenatal clinic booking visit. This is seen by many professionals as a crucial visit for assessing the needs and background of the pregnant women, for planning future care and for health education (Bennett, 1983). However, Methven (1990) notes that professionals vary in their views about the main purpose of the booking visit. Some may see it largely as an information gathering exercise, determined by the need for obstetric case notes, while others may see it as a much broader opportunity to discuss expectations for pregnancy and birth and to plan care accordingly.

The success or otherwise of this visit can influence women's attitudes to the future use of services:

> Whenever she is seen, the woman's response to her initial visit will affect her readiness to take up the care available, to act on advice given, and also to feel secure in seeking answers to her queries (Maternity Services Advisory Committee, 1982, P.8)

McCabe *et al.* (1984) looked at the time spent on the booking visit, and found that for the midwives involved, a very large majority spent 10/30 minutes. However, only 52% were regularly involved in booking visits, with GPs being more involved in some areas. Research in Belfast (McKnight and Merrett, 1986) suggests a difference between midwives and doctors in their approach to the booking visit. They found that more women felt they had had more time to ask questions of the midwife than of the doctor.

The whole experience of the booking visit may also not encourage women, and particularly first-time pregnant women, to feel they can ask questions and find out information. In Perfrement's study (1982) 16% of women said they had not been asked if they had any questions, or had not felt able to ask questions. She suggests that aspects of the organization of the clinic, such as seeing many different staff, militates against asking questions, and that the overall impression of overworked and rushed staff means that parents might feel that questions will hold up the system.

In addition to not feeling able or being encouraged to ask questions, more general feelings about the booking visit will influence women's openness to information and advice. Perfrement's study confirms this view. She reports that 57% of women had largely negative feelings about the booking visit. When interviewed just 2 or 3 days later, only 39% cited the clinic as a source of information about diet, despite 92% having been given written or verbal information about diet at that visit. Perfrement suggests that negative feelings about the clinic could mean that information was not assimilated or recognized by quite a number of women. This may help to explain MacIntyre's (1981) finding that only 16% of women felt they had obtained any information other than the date of confinement or details of benefits at the booking visit.

Several studies report that a significant minority of women attend their first clinic appointment late on in pregnancy. Perfrement (1982) found that 20% did not attend until they were more than 16 weeks pregnant, due largely to delays in GP referral. Chisholm (1989), in a large study in Manchester, found similar late booking rates, with 24% booking after 16 weeks. She also found that there were higher than average late booking rates amongst: teenagers; women over the age of 35; those who were unemployed; and those who moved house during pregnancy. A quarter did not visit their GP to confirm their pregnancy until they were more than 3 months pregnant, and one fifth did not attend antenatal clinic until after Week 20. The implication of both these studies is that GPs have a crucial health education role to play for women who confirm later and then attend antenatal clinics later than average. For some women GPs are the only health professionals with whom they have contact in the first half of pregnancy.

5.3 Antenatal clinic attendance

After the initial booking visit, many women attend antenatal clinics regularly, and it is not uncommon for there to be 12 or more visits during the course of pregnancy. There is plenty of research on women's views about antenatal clinics in general. This consistently shows that women object to long journeys to clinics, long waiting times, lack of continuity of care, the impersonal production-line atmosphere of many clinics and a lack of consistent information and advice (Lupton, 1985; Porter and MacIntyre, 1989). Where women experience a number of these negative aspects of antenatal care, it is likely that their openness to education will be adversely affected.

Much less research has, however, been carried out directly on aspects of education within antenatal care. Graham and McKee (1980) found in a group of first-time mothers, that only 20% said they had learnt anything from clinic attendance. This was despite 90% rating clinic attendance as important. They suggest that a complex interaction of factors related to clinic organization, staff attitudes and women's expectations, tends to work against making the best use of opportunities for learning. MacIntyre (1981) also found that most women said they only got reassurance from antenatal care, and postnatally less than a quarter of mothers rated their antenatal care as having been useful. In contrast, McKnight and Merrett (1986) found in their Belfast study that only around a quarter of women were dissatisfied with the time available for questions and discussion. However, the figures were very much lower for women receiving care at the local health centre or community clinic than at the hospital – a finding replicated by Boyd and Sellers (1982), Lupton (1985) and by Taylor (1986), who found that women particularly valued the quality of communication possible at GP clinics.

Milner (1990) found that 80% of women were satisfied with the amount of information they had received at clinic visits. The most common criticism was a lack of information about test results. MacIntyre (1981), however, found that women criticized the quality of information they were given particularly in relation to anxieties or worries, when general reassurance tended to be given, rather than specific information. Boyd and Sellers (1982) noted that many women had had to rely on primarily written information at the antenatal clinic. They also found that second-time parents felt they had less access to information and advice than first-time parents, because it was assumed they 'knew it all'.

In a large study of women's information needs in pregnancy (Ball, 1989), 24% had felt unable to discuss things fully with health professionals – with more single working-class women and council-house tenants saying this than other groups.

The success of health education on a one-to-one basis depends on a number of complex interaction factors, to do with the setting, time available, perception of need and quality of communication. Where a woman is able to build up a relationship with a health educator who also knows something of her background and need, health education probably stands some chance of success. This suggests that continuity of antenatal care may be important for effective health education. This in turn suggests that local clinic care may offer better opportunities than hospital care. In studying the quality of local GP care, McCabe *et al.* (1984) found that 68% of midwives saw at least half the women on their caseloads four or more times during their antenatal care. Many women were thus experiencing some continuity of care. Lupton (1985) also reports quite high levels of continuity of care, with 50% of women always and 31% usually seeing the same staff. This study also noted that continuity of care was much less common in hospital than community clinics.

In the study by McCabe *et al.* (1984), the midwives who spent the majority of their time on antenatal care and antenatal classes were also found to be highly committed to health education: over 80% of midwives were routinely giving information and advice on a list of 17 topics, which included health, social and emotional aspects of pregnancy (with the exception of sexual relationships). Overall, this suggests that local GP clinic care may provide enhanced opportunities for health education through the commitment of midwives to health education and the greater possibility of continuity of care. However, it is also important to note that where GPs provide more of the routine care than midwives, the opportunities are likely to be poorer. Not only do GPs spend less time with women and give fewer opportunities for questions than midwives, they also tend to have a narrower view of health education (see Section 5.1). McCabe et al. (1984) also found that GPs routinely covered health education less often than midwives, with 80% of GPs routinely covering only 6 out of 17 topics (compared with 16 out of 17 topics for midwives).

The overall approach of staff to their work in the antenatal clinic may also be a significant influence on how far opportunities for education are used. Graham and McKee (1980) note that the clinic routine may tend to be task-focused rather than person-focused, which militates against mothers having open discussion with staff about their pregnancy in general rather than various medical aspects of it. They also found that staff-patient interactions tended to be oriented to physiological and medical aspects of pregnancy, so that women's needs to talk about emotional or subjective aspects of pregnancy tended to be disregarded. This may partly explain their finding that although 57% of women felt there were opportunities to ask questions at the clinic, most actually did not do so.

Finally, it is interesting to note that women themselves may welcome informal opportunities for health education in the clinic. Milner (1987) found that 67% of women felt that the relatively long waiting time could be used to help them, with the most common suggestions being watching videos about pregnancy, childcare and health, and having written information available. The clinic could also be a place where pregnant women talk to one another, and gain support and information from one another, especially as waiting times are long. However, Graham and McKee (1980) found that the organization of the clinic tended to militate against this: only 57% of women in their study said they sometimes talked to other patients, and 92% said they had not made any friends at the clinic.

5.4 Home visiting

Home visits in the antenatal period offer considerable potential for health education. Clinic constraints such as the limited time available, the pressures of the waiting room and the service setting, do not apply in the home where many women are likely to feel more comfortable and in control. The extent of antenatal home visiting by either midwives or health visitors seems to be quite variable. For instance, McCabe et al. (1984) report that two-thirds of health visitors never did any antenatal home visits, whilst most midwives had done at least one home visit in the study period, but generally fairly late on in pregnancy.

Two recent studies have attempted to influence pregnant women's lifestyles, use of health services and pregnancy outcome through a programme of increased support based on home visits. In Leeds (Parker and Ness, 1986) regular antenatal and postnatal home visits were offered to a group of women living in an area of multiple disadvantage. Health outcomes were compared with a similar group of women who received the usual service only. This study claims only small success in being able to influence smoking, diet and drinking habits during pregnancy, and attitudes to breast-feeding and immunization, from an intensive programme of visits and support. In Newcastle (Evans, 1991) a similar project set out to provide support to pregnant women in two multiple-disadvantaged areas, through community midwifery support, providing antenatal home visits, continuity of midwifery care and locally-based special antenatal classes. Detailed evaluation of the project revealed positive effects on smoking and diet, on low birth weight and pre-term delivery, and on general satisfaction with the standard of health services (compared with a non-intervention control group and with previous pregnancies for women in the study group). The reports suggests that the community midwifery practice, with support from home visits, enabled the midwives to gear their antenatal education to the individual social and economic circumstances of the pregnant women. This was reflected in far more women being able to change their behaviour than the control group, which received only standard antenatal advice and education from midwives who did not know them and their circumstances so well.

5.5 The interaction between care and classes

It is important to note from the literature that the provision of quality care can influence the uptake and success of antenatal classes, and vice versa. At the most basic level, women generally receive information and publicity about classes in a care setting, and as already noted in Section 4, the attitudes of staff to classes and the degree to which they both inform women and encourage them to attend affect take-up rates.

Women who receive quality care may also be more inclined to take up classes, perhaps because they are more likely to perceive them as relevant. The Newcastle Community Midwifery Project, for instance (Evans, 1991), showed a dramatic increase in class attendance for a group of particularly disadvantaged women.

Although professionals may tend to separate antenatal classes from antenatal care, and think of antenatal education as synonymous with classes, it is unlikely that this is how pregnant women view these services. Indeed some women are quick to point out that the advice given in classes may differ from that in the clinic or hospital, or that hospital procedures differ from those outlined at classes (see Section 4.2). Not surprisingly, there may also be benefits in the interaction between classes and care, with studies reporting a greater satisfaction with clinic and/or hospital care amongst women who attend classes (for example, Taylor, 1985).

5.6 The roles of different health professionals

The most detailed research on the roles of different health professionals in education within care settings, comes from McCabe *et al*. (1984) in their study of GPs, midwives and health visitors. This study highlighted a number of issues which tended to mean that educational opportunities were being lost. Firstly, they found that GPs were ambivalent about health education and that this could undermine the effectiveness of health visitors and midwives. Secondly, the low level of involvement of health visitors in routine antenatal care meant that their knowledge of social factors and family background rarely influenced the advice and information being given. Thirdly, each professional group tended to underestimate the involvement in the routine health education of the other two groups. This meant that advice on some topics was likely to be repeated, but more importantly, that there was little or no co-ordination, even at local GP level, of the educational side of antenatal care.

A number of studies also suggest that pregnant women generally receive relatively little advice or information from health professionals during pregnancy and, not surprisingly, that they do not see health professionals as a significant source of information. For instance, Madeley *et al*. (1989) found that only 20–22% of women had received information from nurses or hospital doctors on smoking during the antenatal period. Information about alcohol seems even less common, with McKnight and Merrett (1987a) reporting only 4% of women having advice from GPs about drinking, 2% from health visitors and 22% from midwives. Similarly advice about diet was given by midwives to only 33% of women, and by GPs to only 4% of women (McKnight and Merrett, 1987b).

MacIntyre (1981) and Ball (1989) also report that health visitors and midwives are often not seen as a key source of information. Ball (1989) found that working-class women were less likely to see health professionals as a source of information than middle-class women. Adams (1982) found that very few women (1–3%) saw health visitors or midwives as key sources of information, particularly compared with friends, family and books.

These studies provide additional evidence to suggest that health professionals are not using fully or effectively the opportunities they have to provide information to women. It is also worth noting a finding from a small London study, which showed that some women thought that clinic midwives were simply nurses and therefore not an authoritative source of information and advice about pregnancy (Webber and Janzen, 1982). MacIntyre (1981) also reports some confusion amongst women about the professions of the people seen, and that midwives were commonly seen as just nurses, whilst health visitors were confused with social workers, nurses and social security workers. This suggests that clear information about the role of clinic staff might increase the use made of both midwives' and health visitors' health education skills.

5.7 Information and knowledge during pregnancy

A number of studies have looked more widely at women's needs for information and advice during pregnancy. They provide a broad and important context for the work of health professionals.

In a survey in one health district, the information needs of pregnant women were analysed in detail (Mason, 1989). Twice as many first-time mothers (50%) were found to have wanted more information than women who already had babies. Of this group, half were rated initially as already knowing a great deal or quite a lot before pregnancy. This suggests that even if women appear to know much about pregnancy, they will still have significant information needs. In contrast, this study also found that 23% of first-time mothers had neither known much before pregnancy nor wanted to know much more during pregnancy. This suggests that a sizeable minority of women are not very open to education, even as first-time mothers.

The kind of information, advice and support which women want is also important to consider. Mason (1989) found that 61% of first-time mothers had wanted more chances to talk to someone about medical matters or for general advice, support and reassurance. This was the kind of information need mentioned most often as having been unavailable during pregnancy.

In Ball's study (1989) of women's access to information during pregnancy, books, magazines and newspapers were the key information source for 80% of women, followed by husband or partner (75%), other women having a baby (59%) and friends/neighbours (58%). However, she found this pattern altered for women in social class V, for whom husbands and partners were more important, and books and written information very much less important. In this same study, only 6% of women who had attended antenatal classes rated the classes as their most helpful source of information.

Whilst many authors acknowledge the importance of information and advice gained from friends and family, very little research has explored this in detail. In a study in the US on social network advice during pregnancy, 99% of women reported being given advice by friends and family (St Clair and Anderson, 1989). The most common sources of advice were mothers, partners and sisters, and the most common types of advice were to do with hygiene and activity (95% of women), diet (91%), avoidance of harmful substances or practices (85%), and remedies for discomforts in pregnancy (52%). Although most of the advice given was reported as being judged to be sound (i.e. not contradicting current orthodoxy), very often there appeared to be little or no understanding of the basis or reasons for the advice. For a minority of women, outdated medical information was passed on, often by mothers, or anxiety caused by old wives' tales about complications in pregnancy. This research demonstrates the importance of informal sources of information to pregnant women, from people who are trusted and readily accessible in women's everyday lives, and suggests that health professionals need to build on rather than undermine these sources of information.

5.8 Suggestions for improvement

The following ideas are reported in the literature as possible ways of maximizing educational opportunities within antenatal care.

- Greater awareness among women of, and involvement of GPs in, early pregnancy advice, particularly on smoking, drinking, drug use and diet (McKnight and Merrett, 1986; McCabe *et al.*, 1984) but also on the social and emotional aspects of pregnancy, particularly at the confirmation visit (McCabe *et al.*, 1984).
- Increasing the understanding of the importance of continuity of care for effective education (Redbridge and Waltham Forest, 1981; Prince and Adams, 1990).
- Greater involvement of health visitors in antenatal care, including home visits, in order to establish better continuity of care and to enable social factors to influence education (McCabe *et al.*, 1984). Increased antenatal home visits by health visitors, whilst desirable, may be unrealistic (Parker and Ness, 1986).
- Better communication about educational activities within the primary health care team, to reduce repetition of some topics and fill gaps; better clarification of the educational roles of GPs, health visitors and midwives (McCabe *et al.*, 1984).
- Splitting the medical care given at clinics from the educational and support activities and offering an early pregnancy group meeting with a midwife (Perfrement, 1982).
- Increasing professionals' understanding that the whole quality of antenatal care affects education, and that education is not synonymous with antenatal classes. Initiatives to improve access to care are likely to improve access to education (for examples of improvements relating to appointment bookings, transport, provision of play areas, and layout and comfort of waiting areas, see Dowling (1983), Chapter 3).
- Encouraging all practitioners, and particularly GPs, to move away from a medical model of health education, and a prescriptive list of 'dos' and don'ts' in pregnancy, towards a more holistic and socially relevant approach (McCabe *et al.*, 1984).
- Encouraging the development of interactive styles of communication with pregnant women in care settings which take account of existing knowledge and beliefs (McCabe *et al.*, 1984).
- The adoption of more sympathetic and considerate attitudes by care staff which could increase considerably mothers' satisfaction with services (Association of Community Health Councils in England and Wales, 1987).
- Increasing discussion amongst professionals on the details of advice offered, to ensure that conflicting advice is not being given, particularly in relation to diet in pregnancy and infant feeding (Jackson, 1990).
- Providing very practical support (in addition to advice and information) for pregnant women wishing to give up or reduce smoking, in the form of 'Stop-smoking groups' (Parker and Ness, 1986) or individually tailored guidance (Perfrement, 1982).
- Ensuring that clinics are organized so that pregnant women are both encouraged to ask questions and discuss any aspect of their pregnancy, and staff have the information and time to be able to respond (Redbridge and Waltham Forest Area Health Education Service, 1980; Perfrement, 1982; Bennett, 1983; Lupton, 1985; Prince and Adams, 1990).
- Encouraging the understanding and skills of health professionals to adapt information and advice to the needs and circumstances of individual women from a wide range of backgrounds (Graham and McKee, 1980; McCabe *et al.*, 1984).
- Ensuring that the practices promoted in hospital do not conflict with those taught in classes, particularly in relation to breathing and relaxation (Cox, 1985).
- Reviewing the system of GP referrals to antenatal clinics in order to encourage earlier clinic attendance and thus maximize opportunities for education within care (Perfrement, 1982; Webber and Janzen, 1982; Chisolm, 1989).

- Creative use of waiting areas, so that women have access to more written information, and can develop informal contact with other women (Redbridge and Waltham Forest Area Health Education Service, 1980).
- Offering clinic sessions on Saturdays and in the evenings in order to encourage fathers to attend, and to make attendance easier for some working women (Redbridge and Waltham Forest Area Health Education Service, 1980).
- Redirecting priorities and resources for parent education to local areas with high perinatal mortality and morbidity rates (McCabe *et al*., 1984).

Section 6: Postnatal education

The literature on postnatal education is generally less extensive and detailed than for the antenatal period. In particular, there appears to have been much less research on objective outcomes. This section considers the variety of opportunities for education in the postnatal period and assesses how far and how effectively these opportunities are used.

6.1 Care in the immediate postnatal period

For many women, and particularly for first-time mothers, the period directly after the birth of a baby involves two or more days of care from health professionals, in a hospital or GP unit setting. This is a time of adjustment and change, when parents may have a number of different needs, including education, which relate to having given birth and being a parent to a newly born baby.

The Maternity Services Advisory Committee report on postnatal and neonatal care (1985) identified a number of common needs among parents during the immediate postnatal period, which relate to postnatal education:

- Ability to discuss worries and ask questions (Section 2.4 of the Report of the Maternity Services Advisory Committee)
- Ability to talk to other mothers (Section 6.9)
- Advice on the mother's own health, including family planning, rubella and exercise (Sections 2.11 and 2.13)
- Reassurance about emotional reactions and feelings towards the baby (Section 2.26)
- Advice on the needs and care of the baby, including feeding (Sections 2.11 and 2.16)
- Consistent advice and information, which is tailored to individual needs (Section 2.12)

Studies of parents' experiences, however, suggest that some of these needs may not be fully recognized by health professionals, and that the organization of care means that educational opportunities may be missed or reduced in effectiveness.

In a study of women's experiences of postnatal care in hospital, Porter and MacIntyre (1989) found that:

- Contradictory advice was common, especially about breast-feeding and childcare

- Personal matters were often talked about in public, which inhibited proper support and discussion
- Women had few opportunities to ask questions or raise doubts.

The Newham Parents Forum (1988) report also noted that one third of women felt opportunities to ask questions were inadequate. This was perhaps a reflection of the finding that for a minority of women the attitudes of many staff undermined rather than built-up their confidence. Many complaints related to feeding the baby, for which, despite some pressure to breast-feed, there was perceived by some to be a lack of information and practical support.

MacIntyre (1981) also found that women complained about being given conflicting advice on the postnatal ward, or told to adopt overly strict routines for bathing or caring for the baby. However, overall, two-thirds found the parent education they had received to be useful.

One study suggests that parents and professionals differ significantly in how they view parents' needs at this time (Laryea, 1989). Midwives were found to emphasize the biological and medical aspects of motherhood, whilst women tended to emphasize the acquisition of a new social role with social status. This meant that in practice, midwives tended to focus on helping mothers get back to good health so they could take up their responsibilities of infant care. In contrast, mothers expected recognition of their new role but often felt it was ignored in practice. They also felt that their main need was for an understanding of their emotional needs related to this new role. One area where this difference in perspective caused some conflict was in care for the newly born baby. Mothers tended to want to be taught care skills and to learn to decide for themselves when to feed or change their baby. Midwives, however, tended to see their role as deciding what needed to be done when, and then give practical help and support to the mother for feeding or changing.

Parents and professionals may also differ in their views of what is a valued activity. Currell (1990) suggests that many midwives on postnatal wards are task-focused or problem-solving focused. They therefore value helping parents with care tasks or with feeding problems more than talking and listening to them. She notes one study which found that midwives did not approach women on postnatal wards unless there was a specific task to perform.

The above findings suggest that many women experience the postnatal ward as a busy, noisy place in which staff are perpetually in a rush, and in which they adopt a focus on medical aspects of care. Given that some of these findings relate to research carried out five or more years ago, and that there is now an increasing tendency for women to spend less time postnatally in hospital, the prospects for effective parent education in this setting do not seem too bright.

It may be that staff on postnatal wards need opportunities to consider small ways in which their practice could be improved within the constraints of time and resourcing outlined above. They may also need to consider what should be priorities for the small amount of parent education which is possible at this time. This situation also has a knock-on effect on the work of community midwives, who may find themselves increasingly in the position of responding to parents' education and support needs from Day 3 onwards, some of which would formerly have arisen on the postnatal ward.

6.2 Using health services

The main contacts which parents have with the health service in the early months of parenting are with the GP, home visits from midwives and health visitors' and visits to the child health clinic. These all present one-to-one opportunities for the parent and the health professional to discuss concerns, and for parents to be given information and advice. The effectiveness of such work is covered by a considerable volume of general literature on how these services operate. For the purposes of this review, a much smaller number of studies have been selected, which offer particular insight into the educational aspects of these services.

The postnatal clinic may be the first contact a mother has with health professionals outside her home, following discharge from hospital. Porter and MacIntyre (1989) report that a preoccupation in many postnatal clinics with form-filling can lead to women's emotional and social needs being overlooked. She reports that most of the women observed in her study talked about excessive tiredness to the doctors, but this was only acted on medically and if there was thought to be a possibility of anaemia. She contrasts the actual experiences of postnatal clinics with the kind of care and concern women are led to expect from the literature for parents.

A number of studies report that the majority of parents are largely satisfied with their experiences of child health services. For example, Simms and Smith (1984a, b) found dissatisfaction among only 12% of teenage women over visits to GPs, 5% over health visitors' home visits and 20% over child health clinics. Sherratt *et al.* (1991) found 20% of parents critical of clinics or health visitors. One study notes that the groups who found the clinic the most useful and attended most were the first-time mothers and those who breast-fed. In contrast, the experienced mothers and those who bottle-fed found the clinic least useful and attended least often (Graham and McKee, 1980).

Two studies, however, suggest that levels of satisfaction may reduce as the baby gets older: Graham and McKee (1980) found that satisfaction with home visits dropped from 70% of women at 1 month to 56% at 5 months. Similarly satisfaction with the child health clinic dropped from 91% of attenders to 64% between Months 1 and 5. This study raises the interesting question of why the one third of women who express dissatisfaction still continue to attend. Mayall and Foster (1989) suggest that the clinic may be particularly important to isolated women, and serves a social function where mothers can meet and support one another.

In a study of 96 families, Moss *et al.* (1986) found that the proportion of women who had mixed or negative feelings about health visitors rose from 22% at 7 weeks to 42% at 6 months. For clinics the percentage of women with mixed or negative feelings rose from 31% at 7 weeks to 37% at 6 months. Similarly Graham and McKee (1980) found that attendance dropped off more markedly with time for women in social Classes IV and V, who also became more dissatisfied with both the clinic and the health visitor's visits, despite initially rating both services highly. Graham and McKee's study suggests that dissatisfaction with the services related to women being unsure about the services' functions; a feeling that their functions were unimportant or could be more easily met elsewhere; women being made to feel inadequate or embarrassed; and attributing a policing role to the services. The rise in dissatisfaction noted in this study took place almost entirely amongst the working-class group of women.

Graham and McKee also found that a considerable minority of women under-used their GP services because they were uncertain about their child's symptoms and as to whether calling out the GP was warranted or not. This was particularly so for disorders where women were unsure about what symptoms to look for and how significant they were. In contrast, symptoms relating to digestive or respiratory illnesses were fairly easy to detect, and it was for these illnesses that women generally visited or called out the GP. An overall attitude of not wanting to fuss or call on the GP unnecessarily prevailed. Similarly, Sherratt *et al.* (1991) found that, at six months, a mother's primary area of concern was specific medical problems and ailments, and that for these problems they preferred to visit the child health clinic rather than their GP.

It may be that health visitors could also broaden their focus to encompass these medical problems. At present, parents may perceive clinics largely as places to go for checking their baby's weight, for immunization and for general discussion about the baby's health, as suggested in a study by Sherratt *et al.* (1991). However, when they asked parents what worried them most about their baby, medical/physical complaints were commonest (34%) followed by no worries (31%). Growth, feeding and sleeping which are reported elsewhere to be key priorities for health visitors in clinics (Leggett, 1985) were of greatest concern with less than 10% of the parents.

It is also worth noting reports that relatively few parents see the clinic as a key source of written information or a source of social support (Sherratt *et al.*, 1991). Both Sherratt *et al.* (1991) and Moss *et al.* (1986) found that partners and relatives were mentioned as the most useful source of information and advice. In Moss's study, health visitors and clinics were seen as the most useful source of advice by parents only for feeding. Professionals were named as the key source of advice on particular problems to do with feeding, sleeping and behaviour for between only 10% and 27% of parents (with the exception of infant feeding at age six months). GPs were regarded as particularly unimportant to parents, with between only 4% and 8% rating them as the most helpful source of advice.

During the 1980s a significant number of health authorities became involved in a parent education and support initiative known as the Child Development Programme. Specially trained health visitors become first-parent visitors and provide first-time parents with regular home visits, beginning antenatally and continuing at monthly intervals during the baby's first 6 to 8 months of life (Early Childhood Development Programme, 1987a). Anecdotal evidence exists that both parents and health visitors value this programme (Early Childhood Development Programme, 1987b).

Despite the overall high levels of satisfaction reported among parents for child health services, it is important to remember that parents may be reluctant to criticize services, or may have low expectations about how services could be different. Criticisms from a minority are therefore significant as they may provide clues as to how services can be improved for all parents. The main criticisms of relevance to parent education are:

- Advice lacking or too general to be of use
- Irrelevant or conflicting advice
- Poor explanations about procedures and checks at the clinic, leaving women unprepared and not ready to ask questions
- A lack of caring and personal interest taken in the mother and baby
- Patronizing or judgemental staff attitudes
- A lack of time for talking
- A lack of privacy for personal issues to be discussed
- Long waiting times at clinics

(Graham and McKee, 1980; MacIntyre, 1981; Field *et al.*, 1982; Simms and Smith, 1984; Mayall and Foster, 1989)

6.3 Postnatal groups

Four main kinds of postnatal group are reported in the literature, depending on the focus they take.

A focus on baby

These groups focus primarily on childcare and child development. They are often of a fixed length, typically 6–8 weeks, and take a set topic each week for a formal talk from a health professional followed by discussion. Common topics include feeding and weaning, immunization, crying and sleeping problems, general child development, safety, minor illnesses and behaviour problems. These groups are generally set up and led by a health professional and are targeted at mothers in the first months of motherhood. (See for example Bracey and Blythe, 1983.)

A variation on this kind of group is described by Lloyd (1990). In this group mothers were taught skills of interacting and communicating with their young babies in order to increase their understanding of and responsiveness to their babies' needs.

A dual focus on mother and baby

In addition to considering aspects of childcare, some groups also cover the health and well-being of mothers. Common topics here include family planning, breast self-examination, feelings about parenting, and postnatal depression. Again these groups are generally set up and led by health professionals and are of limited duration. Examples are found in McConville (1989); Tether and Hirst (1986); *Health Visitor* (1983).

Several groups are also reported where about half of each session is given over to postnatal exercises, which are followed by informal talks or discussion on health issues relating to mother and baby (Artur and Butt, 1991; Sefi, 1987).

A focus on self-support

The main feature of some groups is that they are largely or entirely parent-led and run, and function first and foremost as support groups. The issues a group considers are determined by the parents, and therefore appear to be much more wide-ranging than the above lists of maternal and child healthcare topics. Equal emphasis is given to social contact, which may include activities and outings, and to practical ways of supporting one another, such as baby-sitting and exchanging baby clothes and toys. Health professionals may be involved in initiating such groups (for example, through organizing a reunion for an antenatal class) or be invited on occasions to talk to a group. Examples are given by Hiskins (1982) and Labrow (1986). The National Childbirth Trust organizes similar self-support groups which may be supported at the outset by a member of an existing group (Wilson, 1986).

A focus on parenting and older and older children

A number of postnatal groups are reported as working with parents after the immediate postnatal period, with a special focus on issues related to parenting. Some of these are targeted at particular groups of parents – often those who are considered to be isolated or in particular need of support because of their social, economic or family circumstances. Willis (1988), for example, describes a support group set up for male single-parents in an inner-city area, and Brown (1989) reports on a parenting group for lone parents. Ruel and Adams (1981) describe a group for parents identified by professionals as experiencing minor parenting problems.

Parents' views

Only five studies of parents' views of postnatal groups were uncovered by this review. Four of these involved getting feedback from mothers who had taken part in groups (Tether and Hirst, 1986; Lloyd, 1983; McConville, 1989; Sefi, 1987), whilst the fifth sought mothers' views on what a group could offer (Smith and Whitehead, 1986).

From this limited amount of small-scale research, there appear to be a number of benefits which parents see in joining a postnatal group:

- Social contact with other mothers with babies
- Sharing experiences, problems and information with other parents
- Meeting a health professional informally

Lloyd (1983) found that these aspects of the groups were valued more highly than specific coverage of health education and baby care topics, which, she suggests, parents may value less than health professionals often suppose. In her study, 96% of mothers in three different groups felt that the group was primarily a social occasion on which to meet other mothers, whilst only 15% thought the group's main purpose was to teach about baby care.

Several other studies, however, suggest that mothers do have an interest in and a need to talk about baby care, but not to the exclusion of other issues. In particular, a mother's own experiences, health and psychological needs seem to be of equal interest and importance to parents (Lloyd, 1983; Smith and Whitehead, 1986). Thus, when mothers in Smith and Whitehead's study were asked what topics a postnatal group should consider, the five most popular topics were feeding (65%), postnatal depression (41%), children's illnesses (39%), general problems including housing and finances (37%), and conflict between a mother's and a baby's needs (30%).

In commenting on the way groups are run, parents appear to value:

- Opportunities for open and in-depth discussion
- An informal structure (although some parents do value occasional formal talks)

Interestingly, in Lloyd's (1983) study which compared three groups with different structures (formal, semi-formal and informal), 100% of mothers in the informal group rated themselves as confident after attending the group, compared with only 44% in the semi-formal group and 22% in the formal group. For some mothers in the formal and semi-formal groups, there were feelings that the group leader had tended to emphasize right and wrong ways of dealing with the care of a baby. Lloyd suggests that this may have undermined rather than increased the mothers' confidence. For other mothers, a time-lag between the finish of one group and the start of the next, meant that by the time they joined a group they had already overcome an initial lack of confidence, which had been felt most acutely in the first 6 weeks after the birth.

Additional comments which parents have made about postnatal groups include:

- The importance of space and facilities for crawling babies (Lloyd, 1983)
- The value placed on active participation in a group by some mothers (Lloyd, 1983; Tether and Hirst, 1986).
- The value of mixing first-time parents with experienced parents (McConville, 1989)

- An over-emphasis by professionals on postnatal contraception (Artur and Butt, 1991)
- A high level of willingness and interest in going to a postnatal group among mothers who do not have access to a group (Curtice, 1989a, b; 89% of mothers in Smith and Whitehead's (1986) study said they would go to a group, and 79% in Cox's study (1985) responded similarly). Section 3 also reported that parents felt they would benefit from self-support groups.

Health professionals' views

Health professionals involved in running postnatal groups tend to report that the groups are attended largely by middle-class, White and well-educated women (Artur and Butt, 1991). There is also often the perception that those who would benefit most from groups are the ones who tend not to come along.

6.4 Parents' needs

The previous three sections have identified a number of needs which parents have in the postnatal period, particularly in relation to the support, information and advice they receive or wish to receive from health professionals. Section 3.6 listed key issues in the postnatal period, as identified by first-time parents. Some additional issues are also discussed in the literature.

Firstly, postnatal depression is an experience which has become increasingly recognized in recent years. Ball (1989) reports that 10% of mothers suffer depression which is severe enough to need psychiatric intervention, whilst a further 10% experience considerable emotional distress and disturbance for weeks or months following the birth. Overall, considerable numbers of women have very specific emotional and support needs, which may go unrecognized by the family, but which the health professional is in a position to both recognize and respond to. Section 3 also highlighted that parents felt that general emotional and psychological needs were largely ignored by health professionals.

Secondly, a study in Liverpool on the health and social support needs of families with a baby in the first year of life, identified three areas of need which were often unmet for parents (Curtice, 1989a, b). These were: learning specific skills; gaining emotional support; and having a testing-board for working out ways of dealing with complex parenting problems with a health dimension. The report suggests that groups which are facilitated properly and provide opportunities to share information and experiences within a safe environment could meet these kinds of needs. Similarly, Billingham (1989) notes that the central issue for many mothers is not knowledge *per se*, but the difficulties of putting knowledge into practice.

Thirdly, one author highlights the importance of fostering the development of mothers as people, and not just as mothers (Billingham, 1989). In providing postnatal education and support, women need opportunities to pursue their own interests and skills unrelated to their role as mothers. No doubt this has a positive contribution to make to their role as mothers, but a contribution which appears to be largely unrecognized or not provided for by health professionals.

Fourthly, the research reported in Section 3 highlighted two additional postnatal needs which may not be tackled within the health services. These are concerns about body image and anxieties about conflicting advice and how to deal with it effectively.

6.5 Parents' and professionals' perspectives on postnatal education

A recent small-scale qualitative study on parents' and professionals' perspectives of child health care raises some important issues for postnatal education (Mayall and Foster, 1989). Although the study looked at mothers with a first child aged 21 months, the general findings and issues raised are also likely to be significant in the earlier postnatal period.

The mothers in this study saw it as their role to judge when to seek advice from health professionals, and did so having weighed information from a range of informal sources and from their own knowledge of their child. When mothers did seek advice, they wanted time to talk and to be listened to, as well as to have a non-directive discussion between equals. However, amongst the health visitors in the study only 13% appeared to believe in this kind of equal partnership as a model for health education. A further one third combined the idea of dialogue with moving mothers in the 'correct' direction, whilst over half felt they should be trying to change mothers' behaviours, albeit using a covert style. For those who sought behaviour change particular emphasis was placed on the need for a good relationship to enable mothers to be open to advice.

In the same study, differences between parents' and professionals' perspectives on the role of a parent were also found. The mothers stressed equally the need to both care for their children through love, play, talk, teaching and so on, and to provide for them by having adequate housing, income and social life. Most, though not all, of the health visitors, however, gave much less weight to the provision of material resources, which they saw as background factors. They tended to focus instead on promoting good childcare practices and relationships (Mayall and Foster, 1987).

What this study reveals is a disparity between parents and professionals, and perhaps an explanation for why parent education may fail, or why parents do not fully use child health services. It points to the need for professionals to understand parents' perspectives, and to design approaches to parent education which build on rather than contradict these perspectives. It also points to the need for professionals to actively recognize how parenting and choices about parenting are closely bound up with access to resources.

6.6 Suggestions for improvement

The following suggestions for improvement are based on the research findings reviewed earlier in this section.

Care in the immediate postnatal period

- More opportunities for unhurried discussions with health professionals and chances to ask questions.
- Ensuring that discussions about personal and sensitive matters take place in privacy, so that parents feel free to talk openly.
- Greater recognition of the emotional needs of mothers, and active encouragement from health professionals to talk about feelings.
- Encouraging parents to make their own decisions about the care of the baby, with the support of a health professional – thus developing the confidence and skills they will need once they return home.
- Greater recognition of the needs of multiparous women, that they do not 'know it all'.

Child health services

- Ensuring that adequate opportunities are provided for unhurried questions and discussion.
- Recognition of the social function of clinics in facilitating contact amongst women and actually promoting this – for example, through the provision of play areas and the layout of waiting areas.
- Recognizing the importance parents attach to defining their own needs and choosing when to ask for advice or information.

Postnatal groups

- Increasing the availability and accessibility of postnatal groups.
- Recognizing the need for postnatal groups both soon after the birth, and later on when the child is 4–6 months old.
- Promoting groups which are informal in nature and primarily follow parents' expressed needs.
- Focusing group activities on the application of knowledge to everyday life, rather than knowledge *per se*.
- Placing equal emphasis on the interests and experiences of both child and parents.

Overall

- Greater recognition of the emotional and psychological needs of parents.
- Attempting to reduce the amount of conflicting advice given by health professionals, and helping parents to deal more effectively with conflicting advice.
- Wherever possible and when asked by parents, offering concrete and realistic information rather than more general reassurance.

- Providing parents with practical information and support over childhood ailments and illnesses, and the appropriate use of health services.
- Acknowledging the structural factors which influence child and maternal health – such as housing and income.
- Giving greater consideration to the needs of fathers and their roles in parenting, in the ways services are organized and targeted.
- Improving access to general postnatal care and clinics, which itself helps improve access to education in these settings (see suggestions for antenatal clinics in Section 4.8).
- Acknowledging that supporting parents in developing their own interests and education will have a positive impact on their role as parents.

Section 7: Special provision and special needs in parent education

7.1 Young parents

Young parents are considered to have some special needs, both antenatally and postnatally. The most common points made in the literature about young parents and particularly young women are:

- Higher than average rates of obstetric and postnatal complications (Slager-Earnest et al., 1987; NCOPF, 1979)
- Under-use of health services: late booking for antenatal care is more common (Russell, 1988) and attendance at antenatal classes less common than for older women (see Section 4.1)
- Poor housing and low income (Simms and Smith, 1986)
- Likelihood of being single parents (Mills, 1990), which itself may be associated with lack of support and inadequate housing and income levels
- Likelihood of experiencing more depression and anxiety, because pregnancy and parenting induces a state of dependency at a time when increased independence is desired (Lineberger, 1987); or because of isolation and poverty (Simms and Smith, 1984a, b)
- Particular likelihood of being influenced by the responses and decisions of other adults around them, because they are less likely to be financially, emotionally and physically independent (NCOPF, 1979)
- Isolation from friends and family, particularly if the pregnancy is unplanned or the woman is very young (NCOPF, 1979)
- Low levels of self-esteem (although the research evidence for this is contradictory) (Lineberger, 1987).

Several authors comment that younger teenagers (aged 16 and under) are likely to experience more of the factors listed above than older teenagers, although this is not always so where the immediate family provides practical support (NCOPF, 1979).

It is also worth noting that young parents seem, from the literature, to be considered to be an 'at risk' group. Whilst this may be the dominant view, particularly amongst service providers, several studies of teenage parents suggest that there are both negative and positive aspects to being a young mother, and that there is such variety in their experiences, that they cannot be considered so simply to be 'at risk' (Phoenix, 1991; McRobbie, 1991). Indeed, Sadler (1988) notes that the vulnerability of young parents arising from their social and economic circumstances and their emotional development can be seen either as a liability or an asset. As an asset, it may be a time of need when young people are particularly open to and ready for supportive parent education.

Antenatal care

A number of studies highlight that young women often make less use of antenatal care than other groups of women. Perhaps most significant is that many confirm their pregnancy and book for antenatal care much later on in their pregnancy (Simms and Smith, 1984a, b; Chisholm, 1989). Both studies found that more than a quarter of teenagers did not consult their doctors to confirm the pregnancy until they were more than three months pregnant. For many, this was because they did not realize they were pregnant, but for others it was due to fear or embarrassment, and for a few because they feared being talked into abortion (Simms and Smith, 1989a, b).

For these young women who confirm their pregnancy late, the GP has an important role to play, particularly as the late confirmation also tends to lead to late attendance at the antenatal clinic.

Simms and Smith found that 20% of teenage women visited the clinic for the first time after the 20th week of their pregnancy. Higher than average numbers of young (under 17) and single women were also found to be late attenders – in fact, half of the single women were late attenders. Women who are both young and single may therefore miss out on opportunities for parent education in the first part of their pregnancy. This makes it important for health professionals to use any opportunities for education in antenatal care as effectively as possible. Simms and Smith (1984a, b), however, report that 20% of their teenage women were not satisfied with their antenatal care, largely because of waiting times and lack of information. In a survey of antenatal care in one health district, Mason (1989) found that the younger women (in this case, aged under 25) were the group least likely to have talked to midwives or doctors for advice during pregnancy. Similarly, Ball (1989) found that single women experienced more difficulties in obtaining the information they wanted about pregnancy, than married women.

The NCOPF report on pregnancy among schoolgirls notes that young and particularly single women may be reluctant to go to antenatal clinics alongside older, married women, and therefore recommends separate provision which can be geared to young women's particular needs. In a recent survey of 117 maternity units, Minns (1990) found that only 6 (5%) provided separate antenatal clinics for young parents. Nunnerley (1985) describes one such example of separate clinic provision which involves continuity of care, access to a social worker and health visitor, and opportunities for women to talk informally to one another and to health professionals.

Antenatal classes

Given that young women may receive less antenatal care than other women, opportunities for education through antenatal classes become particularly significant. However, as Section 4.1 reports, young women are often very underrepresented at classes. The main reasons for this, given by the professionals interviewed for this review, are:

- Lacking confidence with older women
- Feeling stigmatized if they are single, and intimidated when other women attend with partners
- Not feeling able to ask questions
- Not having their special needs addressed (such as benefits and housing advice; coping on a low income)

In recognition of both these difficulties and the special circumstances and needs of young women, special antenatal classes are provided in quite a number of areas. In a recent survey of 117 maternity units, 37% were found to provide separate antenatal classes for teenage women (Minns, 1990).

These special classes commonly share a number of features:

- An emphasis on developing friendships and support networks (for example, Stringer 1986; Watson 1991)
- An informal approach, with health professionals adopting a low profile in the group (for example, Todd, 1988; Watson, 1991)
- Replacing a planned programme with sessions based on topics the women themselves choose (eg. Todd, 1988; Leigh, 1987)
- Encouraging the sharing of views and experiences (eg. Stringer, 1986)
- Reducing the time spent on breathing and relaxation (eg. Todd, 1988)
- Providing social and fun activities as well as group sessions (eg. Stringer 1986)
- Personal contact through home visits to encourage attendance (eg. Watson, 1991) or collecting women from home to classes (eg. Stringer, 1986)
- Providing antenatal care at the same time (eg. Leigh, 1987)
- Providing benefits and welfare advice (eg. Bristol Evening Post, 1989; Watson, 1991) and access to a social worker (eg. Minns, 1990)
- Mixing together pregnant women with those who have recently had a child, to share experiences (eg. Billingham 1989; Minns 1990)
- Meeting in community premises rather than Health Service premises (eg. Stringer, 1986) or providing parent education within schools to pregnant women (NCOPF, 1979)

Taken together, these features of classes amount to a significantly different approach to antenatal classes from those generally provided.

Resources

Finally, it is worth noting some dissatisfaction among health professionals about the lack of appropriate written and audiovisual materials for young women. Minns's (1990) survey found only three maternity units (out of 117) used materials designed to appeal especially to young parents.

7.2 **Parents from ethnic minority groups**

Ethnic minority groups are also considered to have some special needs antenatally and post natally, which are relevant to parent education. Thse relate to:

- Higher than average rates of perinatal mortality and morbidity, stillbirth and congenital problems (particularly amongst women born in Pakistan and the Caribbean)
- Low uptake of health services: late confirmation of pregnancy, late booking for antenatal care and poor uptake of antenatal classes
- Reduced access to good quality housing and employment
- Reduced access to information and support due to language and communication barriers
- Experience of individual and institutionalized racism, both generally and within the health service.

(Townsend and Davidson, 1982; Pearson, 1985; Whitehead, 1987; Firdous and Bhopal, 1989)

Sources of information

Overall the studies reviewed suggest that some ethnic minority groups may have reduced access to information about pregnancy and parenting, particularly if they have little or no English.

In a study of Asian women in Birmingham, Jain (1985) found that the most important source of advice about care in pregnancy was the GP, who for most of the women was Asian. However, one third of the women asked nobody for advice and this rose to 43% for the Pakistani Muslim women. For some women, having a male GP may deter them from seeking advice and discussing their pregnancy, and particularly the emotional side of pregnancy (Jain, 1985; McCabe et al., 1984). Interestingly, McCabe et al. (1984) also found that GP receptionists had an important role to play in giving advice and information to Asian women, particularly on sensitive issues which the Asian GPs reported finding it hard to broach.

In a survey in one Health District, almost half of all pregnant Asian women were found to have wanted more information during pregnancy, irrespective of how much they knew before the pregnancy or whether or not it was their first baby (Mason, 1989). This suggests that many women were going through pregnancy with needs for information unmet.

For the Asian women in the Newham study, who were Muslim, Hindu and Sikh (Woollett and Dosanjh-Matwala, 1990a, b) leaflets from the hospital were the source of information mentioned most often (94% of women). These leaflets were in English and some Asian languages. This contrasts somewhat with Jain's finding that less than 5% of women were offered written information in an Asian language (although this may be accounted for by Jain's study being undertaken in the early 1980s, when considerably less information was available in languages other than English, and before the Asian mother and baby campaign).

Research on the Health Education Authority's *Pregnancy Book* (1989) amongst eight different minority groups found that one third of women had not seen the book. Chinese, Turkish and Bengali women had least access to the book, with 50% not having seen it. The main reasons for not receiving a copy of the book were supplies running out and hospital staff and linkworkers prioritizing those women who could read English well. This research however, pointed out that the women who did not receive the book were also those who had least access to other sources of information and could gain much by looking at the photographs and drawings. This was particularly so for Vietnamese and Bengali women.

The quality of written information in other languages was criticised by health professionals in the study by McCabe *et al.* (1984). Some leaflets were felt to be too middle class in the lifestyles depicted and advice offered, and written in language many women would not normally use. There was also concern expressed that health workers had little choice in the written information provided in languages other than English, and were not easily able to assess how useful or appropriate it was for their own local patients.

Linkworkers also have a key role to play in increasing many women's access to information during pregnancy, labour and as a parent. An evaluation of the Asian mother and baby campaign concluded that linkworkers helped to improve one-to-one communication between patients and carers, thus reducing stress levels for both parties and providing emotional support to pregnant women (Rocheron and Dickinson, 1990). This study also noted some confusion about the role of linkworkers, and that different aspects of their role could sometimes be in conflict – in particular, how far they were interpreters; advocates for women; and advocates for challenging racism within the service which employed them.

Some research reports that, despite linkworker schemes becoming more common, there are still gaps in the service provided, because of:

- Too great a demand for the available linkworkers (Jain, 1985; McCabe *et al.*, 1984)
- Linkworkers being expected, unrealistically, to be fluent in several languages (Jain, 1985)
- Linkworkers not being available to ethnic minority groups whose numbers are relatively small (Jain, 1985; Cities Research Unit, 1989).

Consequently, some women have to rely on husbands or relatives to accompany them and interpret for them on hospital and clinic visits. Jain (1985) suggests that this may mean some women are inhibited by the person accompanying them from discussing concerns fully with health professionals. McCabe *et al.* (1984) also note that relatives may interpret rather than translate, or may fail to translate accurately complex medical or health information with which they are not themselves familiar.

On a similar theme, Woollett and Dosanjh-Matwala (1990) note that women who had little English had much reduced access to information because they have smaller support networks, are generally less well informed, are less able to make use of information provided at clinics, and have fewer chances to discuss concerns with medical staff.

Finally, Firdous and Bhopal (1989) confirm the view that some Asian women have less initial knowledge about reproductive issues than non-Asian women. They found that for a group of mostly Pakistani Muslim women with little English, knowledge about medical procedures such as amniocentesis was particularly poor. Knowledge about other matters such as breast-feeding, ultrasound and iron/vitamin supplements was, however, as good as amongst non-Asian women.

Antenatal care

Whilst it is generally held that women from ethnic minority groups tend to be late in both confirming their pregnancies and booking at antenatal clinics, the research evidence for this is somewhat mixed. Jain (1985), for instance found that around half of the Asian women in the Birmingham study confirmed their pregnancies before 10 weeks. This was however, less common for the Bangladeshi women. Slightly later booking for antenatal care was found amongst Asian women by Firdous and Bhopal (1989) whilst Chisholm (1989) found no difference between ethnic groups in a large study in Manchester, likewise Rocheron and Dickinson (1990) in the districts evaluated for the Asian mother and baby campaign.

Another common belief is that women from ethnic minorities tend to miss more antenatal appointments, but again the evidence does not fully support this belief. Both Jain (1985) and Woollett and Dosanjh-Matwala (1990) found that very few women missed appointments. Jain, however, found that Bangladeshi and Pakistani women were more likely to do so, though still only a small minority. This may be partly accounted for by the fact that less than 10% of the Bangladeshi women felt the interpreter at the clinic was reliable.

The organization of clinics, and particularly the long waiting times, may reduce the accessibility of ethnic minority women to information and support – Woollett and Dosanjh-Matwala (1990) suggest that long waiting times might deter women from bringing friends or relatives to accompany them to the clinic to act as interpreters.

Antenatal classes

As already reported earlier (4.1 and 4.3) women from ethnic minority groups, and particularly those needing interpreters, rarely attend antenatal classes. For the professionals interviewed for this review, the barriers to ethnic minority women attending classes were:

- Lack of interpreters
- Lack of written information about classes in languages other than English
- Perceived differences in cultural traditions, moral standards and childcare practices, which made it hard for English health professionals to teach classes
- Lack of parent educators from ethnic minority groups.

Several people also felt that the style of classes, when run for Asian groups, tended to be more formal and didactic, because health professionals felt that this was what the women expected. However, such an approach meant that the sessions were very knowledge-based and tended to ignore the social and emotional aspects of pregnancy.

Postnatal education

Newham Parents Forum (1988) reports that, on the postnatal ward, most of the Afro-Caribbean women felt they had had inadequate opportunities to ask questions (compared with an overall figure of one third). About half of the Asian women had also felt they were badly treated on the ward because of their race. Complaints included being ridiculed or staff being impatient or patronizing, particularly to those who did not speak much English. Poor quality of care such as this inevitably affects the openness of women to education, and their perception of health professionals as sources of information, advice and support.

From a slightly different angle, one study suggests that, whilst Asian fathers are often as involved in the birth and hospital as non-Asian fathers, they may play a much less active and supportive role postnatally at home (Woollett and Dosanjh-Matwala, 1990). Female friends and relatives were found in this study to be particularly important at this time, but a significant minority (18%) of women who were living in more nuclear families lacked this support, and experienced considerable isolation.

Mayall and Foster's (1989) study also highlights that women who had arrived recently in Britain relied more heavily on health workers than other women, because they lacked support from near relatives and friends. They also found that women from ethnic minority groups tended to experience problems such as poor housing, low income and a lack of day-care facilities, along with feelings of isolation and experiences of hostility and racism. The authors note, however, that, although health visitors acknowledged the importance of these structural influences on health, they felt powerless to change them, and ended up trying to influence individual behaviours which the women usually lacked the power to change.

Local initiatives

In recent years, a variety of local initiatives has developed to increase the access of ethnic minority groups to health education during pregnancy, and better quality maternity care. In a directory of local projects compiled by the Maternity Alliance in 1985, the following kinds of initiative are noted:

- Antenatal classes targeted at specific ethnic or language groups and adapted to meet specific needs
- English language teaching relating to pregnancy and maternity services
- Communication skills training for health professionals
- Interpreter and linkworker schemes
- Community-based advocates and advice schemes.

English language teaching schemes seem to be particularly common, and were included in fifteen out of the thirty-four projects listed. However, whilst women should have access to such schemes, the schemes are unlikely to be able to meet many of the women's needs. Most women's primary need during pregnancy is for information, support and services relevant to their own circumstances, with an ability to speak English very much a subsidiary part of this.

Additional suggestions to improve access to parent education include:

- Antenatal classes based in local community settings with which women are already familiar
- Greater availability of paid language interpreters, who are familiar with parent education issues
- Co-teaching of classes and groups around health professionals and bilingual outreach or community workers, or ESL teachers
- Wider publicity about existing antenatal classes and postnatal groups which are bilingual or in a mother tongue
- Visits to maternity suites accompanied by language support workers
- Availability of community advice and benefits available at antenatal and postnatal clinics
- Racism awareness and cultural awareness training for health professionals
- Availability of female GPs and hospital doctors, and particularly female doctors from ethnic minority groups
- Appointment of more health workers from ethnic minority groups
- In-service training and peer support for health professionals on antenatal health and race issues (McCabe et al., 1985; Pearson 1985; Munro, 1988)

To conclude, women from ethnic minority groups appear to share a similar reduced access to parent education to young women. Certain groups, however, also experience a considerable language and communication barrier, along with racism, which may affect education in quite subtle ways.

7.3 **Fathers and partners**

Three themes emerge from the literature on the educational needs of fathers and partners:

- To increase their knowledge and understanding of pregnancy in order to support their partner
- To prepare for being a supporter during labour
- To explore and prepare for their role as a father.

An overall emphasis on fathers' sharing in pregnancy and parenting is evident both in literature for parents (Meerabeau, 1987) and in the professional literature about parents. However, practice does not seem adequately to reflect this view about the role of fathers.

Access to education

The literature review failed to reveal any reports or articles about the role of fathers and partners in antenatal care. By not taking part, or being encouraged to do so, they lacked access to a potentially significant source of information and advice. Hanson and Bozett (1986) note that the organization of clinics and their opening times do little to encourage men to attend.

This means that participation in antenatal classes is the only formal educational opportunity for fathers provided by the health service. However, as reported in 4.1, provision is patchy and uptake rates are low. Not surprisingly, then, several studies have found that men rely mostly on their own partner, television and books for information about pregnancy and parenting (McKee 1980; Thompson, 1982).

Antenatal classes

Not only is there far from universal provision of classes for fathers and partners, but what is provided tends not to meet their needs, by focusing largely on their role in labour and birth (see 4.2). Even when men attend the full set of antenatal classes with their partners, their needs may not be fully met, because the classes often tend:

- To be geared to women's needs and experiences
- To be led by women
- Not to address men's needs and interests directly.
  (Pearson and O'Brien, 1987)

Men may also find it hard to participate in a class alongside women, because they see pregnancy as an exclusively female experience and because it may be hard to express feelings in front of their partners and other women (Fenton,

1987). Several authors stress the particular emotional needs of fathers, who may have less day-to-day chances than women to talk over their fears and hopes with friends (Fenton, 1987; Holden, 1990; see Section 3.5).

These observations have led to some practitioners setting up special classes for fathers only (Gregory, 1981; Fenton, 1987). Taubenheim and Silbernagel (1988) describe a support group for fathers consisting of five weekly sessions co-led by a male and female leader. The sessions explored the role of fathers, their feelings about being a parent, and strategies to cope with lifestyle changes.

The inclusion of fathers in antenatal classes also emerged as an area of debate amongst the professionals interviewed for this review. A number felt that having men in a group altered the dynamics in such a way that some women were inhibited from participating fully. This meant that women's needs were not fully met, and, for some, this was seen as the over riding priority. Several people also noted that rooms might not be large enough to accommodate partners, or that groups became too large for good discussion. If more partners were encouraged to come to classes in some areas, it was felt that staff would not be able to cope with the demand.

Finally, it is interesting to note that there is evidence that, if fathers are encouraged during pregnancy to take an active parenting role, this can help to reduce the susceptibility of women to depression after the birth (Holden, 1990).

Postnatal education

Much of the literature notes a distinct lack of education, support and services for fathers in their role as parents. Henderson and Brouse (1991) found that in the first three weeks after the birth, fathers typically go through a pattern of feeling disruption, discomfort and exclusion, and the need to become more involved with the baby. For many these feelings were not what they had anticipated, and during this time their partner was their only source of support (although she too was experiencing difficulties in making the transition to being a mother).

Fathers rarely play more than a support role in hospital, and after this rarely or never have direct contact with health professionals over their baby (Moss, 1986; Mayall and Foster, 1989). Mayall and Foster found they were rarely mentioned as significant by either doctors or health visitors, and that health visitors tended to perceive women as the main care-givers and as the target for their work, even when that included getting mothers to influence fathers' behaviour. They suggest, for the future, more flexible opening hours for clinics and surgeries so that working fathers can become more involved; group work for men on their role as fathers; and consideration of how the needs of male single parents can be met. Moss (1986) also suggests that fathers should be considered primarily as new parents postnatally, with equal rights, interests and obligations towards their children and the health services, and that this should be reflected in the way these services are provided.

7.4 **Experienced parents**

Parents who have already had one or more children still have educational and support needs. The small amount of literature on this topic suggests that women need to:

- Review and share their previous birth experiences
- Have up-to-date information about the practices of the place where they will give birth
- Revisit and practise relaxation and breathing skills
- Consider how a new baby will fit into the family – in particular, coping with an existing child's reactions and coping with fatigue.
  (Williams and Booth, 1984; MacDonald 1987; Macer-Wright, 1987)

Both Macer-Wright and MacDonald stress the importance of assessing what a group of experienced parents needs to learn rather than imposing a programme, and the importance of women sharing their experiences with one another. This contrasts with some current practice with first-time parents which is more directed by professionals and has more emphasis on information-giving. Such an approach is inappropriate with parents who have already experienced pregnancy, birth and parenting.

The importance of providing play or crèche facilities in order to encourage experienced parents to attend antenatal classes, was emphasized by the professionals interviewed for this review and in the uptake studies reviewed in 4.1.

Several studies reviewed in earlier sections suggest that experienced parents' needs are neither recognized nor met in practice:

- They may be invited less often to antenatal classes (Perkins, 1979)
- They are assumed to have been to classes in a previous pregnancy but often have not (Perkins, 1979)
- They may be given advice and information on a one-to-one basis by health professionals less frequently than first-time parents (Boyd and Sellers, 1982; see also 3.5)
- Health advice from professionals may not take account of the presence of existing children – for example, advice on taking rest during pregnancy (Boyd and Sellers, 1982, see also 3.5)
- Child health services are often geared more to the needs of first-time parents (Graham and McKee, 1980; Curtice, 1989).

7.5 **Parents with disabilities**

The needs of parents with disabilities in relation to parent education are very poorly documented. This review located only two British articles and one book on this subject, and therefore draws also on literature from North America. Current British textbooks fail to mention either how to adapt teaching methods or the content of parent education in order to cater for the needs of parents with disabilities (also reported by McEwan Carty et al. (1990) in a review of North American textbooks).

The literature suggests that parents with disabilities have less access than other parents to written and verbal information, for a number of reasons:

- Lack of relevant and accessible written literature
- Poor access to health service premises, prohibiting full use of the services on offer
- Lack of encouragement from health professionals to go to classes or learn exercises
- Negative attitudes of health professionals which prevent women from asking questions and asking for support
- Health professionals poorly informed about the impact of disabilities on pregnancy, birth and parenting, and about practical aids and support agencies available
- Antenatal classes not adapted in content or teaching methods used.
  (Rotherham, 1989; Jackson, 1990; Campion, 1990)

A review by Conine *et al.* (1986) in Canada of the attitudes of childbirth educators in one local area, found that many were aware of the particular needs of parents with disabilities but felt that it was the responsibility of others to meet these needs (other disabled people, specialist agencies, or other health professionals). They suggest a three-pronged approach to improving this situation: provision of better information about parenting and disability; provision of specialist help through a resource centre; training for educators. Campion (1990) provides a useful checklist for health professionals on practical steps in communicating with and teaching women with different disabilities.

McEwan Carty *et al.* (1990) and Campion (1990) both note that parents with disabilities may feel very isolated because of their special needs, and will benefit greatly from being put in touch with other women in a similar position. Prince and Adams (1990) suggest that women with disabilities should be able to go to a special support group organized within the antenatal care system.

Overall, it appears that the needs and experiences of parents with disabilities are largely neglected in relation to parent education, and that this is an area for which there have so far been few initiatives or resources developed.

7.6 Women with multiple pregnancies

Women expecting to have a multiple birth may miss out on antenatal classes because they often deliver early. They also have some special needs: worrying that labour will be longer and more painful, and worrying about how to cope with two or more babies practically, emotionally and financially. There may also be worries about the reactions of other family members, and the impact of multiple pregnancy on the mother's own health. Spillman (1990) notes that parents may have ambivalent feelings about multiple pregnancy and may feel unable to ask for advice or information. This is particularly so when access to written information on multiple births is limited (as in most general antenatal literature).

One report details a special antenatal class for mothers expecting twins, which starts at 22 weeks and is designed to cover their special needs (Holmes, 1988).

Particular needs may be to look carefully at the father's/partner's role, and to consider ways of coping by 'cutting corners' (Spillman, 1990). Postnatal support groups may also be available in some areas through local branches of the Twins' Club.

7.7 Parents living in temporary accommodation

One author reports on the needs of pregnant women living in temporary hotel accommodation (Hibbitt, 1990). Antenatal classes did not attract this group of women largely because health issues related to pregnancy and childbirth were very low on their list of priorities. They also felt that other women in the classes would ostracize them and that the information given would not be relevant to their own living situations. Based on the needs identified by the women themselves, a regular drop-in session was established to provide pregnancy tests, equipment and clothes exchange, benefits and housing advice, exercise, and referrals to other support agencies.

7.8 Adoptive parents

A recent article notes the special needs of parents who are expecting to adopt a baby (Stewart and Ring, 1991). Adoptive parents lack the usual nine-month preparation period of pregnancy, and often have to confront issues about what they tell to whom about the baby. During the placement period prior to the adoption order, they may be unwilling to discuss difficulties for fear of being seen as unable to cope. Although adoptive parents may be invited to antenatal classes, they generally seem to decline to attend, since most are infertile couples, and therefore not comfortable with a group of pregnant women. Stewart and Ring describe a special parentcraft group for adoptive parents in Bristol, designed to meet the special needs outlined above, and to foster mutual support.

7.9 Is class important?

From the literature it is not immediately obvious that class is a significant issue in parent education. There are few reports of work with particular groups, based primarily on class. However, from this review, it is apparent that working-class women, and particularly those in socio-economic groups D and E, have some different experiences and concerns relating to their class:

- Lower uptake of antenatal classes (see Section 4.1) and postnatal groups (see Section 7.3)

- Less access to the basic resources needed for health and poorer access to health services (Townsend and Davidson, 1982)
- Increased levels of stress during pregnancy due to factors such as low income, poor housing, poverty
- Higher than average levels of neonatal and perinatal mortality (Townsend and Davidson, 1982).

In the previous sections, a number of studies reported significant findings relating to class, which are relevant to parent education. In summary, working-class women may tend, more than middle-class women, to:

- Have fewer criticisms and be generally more appreciative of antenatal classes (Taylor, 1985)
- Feel unable to discuss their pregnancy fully with health professionals (Ball, 1989)
- Reject standard advice as irrelevant to their circumstances, particularly if living on a low income (Evans, 1991)
- Be unlikely to see health professionals as a key source of advice and information during pregnancy (Ball, 1989)
- Attach particular importance to advice from husbands and partners and relatively less importance to books, newspapers and magazines (Ball, 1989)
- Benefit more from parent education, because initial knowledge levels tend to be significantly lower (although findings on this are somewhat contradictory – see 6.2)
- Need social support and individually tailored advice to encourage behaviour change during pregnancy and as a parent (Evans, 1991; Parker and Ness, 1986)
- Become more dissatisfied with health visitor advice as the baby becomes older, and use child health clinics less often (Moss, 1986).

It is also important to note that class and/or socio-economic status are often important aspects in the experiences of women from ethnic minority groups and young parents.

Finally, one author raises a particularly significant issue which is remarkably absent from the literature. McIntosh (1989) suggests that working-class women have a different perspective on pregnancy and childbirth from middle-class women. His study of eighty working-class women found that they placed little value on childbirth itself, and rarely saw it as the 'birth experience' middle-class women may look forward to. They tended to see it much more as a medical procedure and expected to have pain relief or other interventions. McIntosh suggests that working-class women have more anxieties and needs for reassurance about the medical aspects of labour than middle-class women. Most expected it to be a frightening and negative experience, and, for some, there was a distinct lack of prior information about the interventions they did experience.

This study is significant because it raises the question of whether the current emphasis, particularly in classes, on breathing, relaxation, choice and control in labour is relevant only to middle-class women.

7.9 Resources for parent education

Textbooks

Two main texts for practitioners were published in the period covered by this review: *Antenatal education: guidelines for teachers* (Williams and Booth, 1985) and *Antenatal teaching: a guide to theory and practice* (Wilson, 1990). Both these books contain a lot of detailed information about pregnancy, labour and postnatal baby care, and include ideas for how this can be presented and discussed in classes. The planning and preparation of classes is also included, along with teaching and learning methods.

Additional texts focus on particular aspects of classes. *Teaching active birth* (Robertson, 1988) contains information and exercises on active approaches to birth.

Antenatal group skills training: a manual of guidelines (Murphy-Black and Faulkner, 1988) concentrates on planning and preparation, and the skills involved in running group sessions.

Resource manuals

Two manuals have been published which provide stimulus materials and methods for practitioners to use in antenatal classes and postnatal groups.

Working together. A health resource pack for working with groups (Billingham, 1990), contains sections on pregnancy and childbirth, caring for children, and women as mothers, with ideas for participatory activities on a range of specific topics. Teaching methods and the organization of group work are also covered in an introductory section.

The *Pipsi activity pack* (Green and Reavill, 1989) contains a wide selection of activities on pregnancy, labour, parenting, infant feeding, child development, and includes brief details about planning, teaching and evaluating participative group work.

Preparing for the new life (McCutcheon, 1991) is an information pack for health professionals on preconception care and education.

The child development programme (see 6.2) produces a selection of information resources, including cartoons for use by first-parent visitors with parents, on a range of child health and development topics. Available only to those who have undergone the training.

Leading antenatal classes. A practical guide (Priest and Shott, 1991) is a book for professionals, which combines some of the information usually covered in textbooks with practical activities for use in classes. It also includes detailed discussion of the aims of classes, and practicalities of planning, teaching and evaluation.

Maternity care for the deaf (Kelsall et al., 1990) is an information pack for midwives which outlines what midwives need to do to make services accessible to women with hearing impairments. The book includes a section on parentcraft teaching.

A good sign goes a long way – The experience of deaf mothers (Lewis, 1991) is a pamphlet detailing deaf women's experiences of maternity care, and ideas for improvements.

Books for parents

There is a very wide range and large number of books available that are written for parents on many aspects of pregnancy and parenting. These may be used by professionals as sources of additional information. The most widely accessible books for first-time parents and health professionals are probably the *Pregnancy Book* (Health Education Authority, 1984) and *Birth to Five* (Health Education Authority, 1989). These cover issues which appear to be largely excluded from the publications aimed at professionals, and may therefore also be of use to practitioners.

The Baby Challenge: a handbook on pregnancy for women with a physical disability (Campion, 1990) covers a range of disabilities and their practical implications for pregnancy and birth, as well as looking at how to get the best out of health services.

Relaxation classes (Two Can Project, 1984) is a short publication aimed at women with a hearing impairment. A series of simple line drawings, accompanied by the appropriate signs, show relaxation exercises, breathing, labour positions and the stages of labour.

Your baby, your choice. A guide to planning your labour (Maternity Alliance, 1990) is a practical resource aimed at helping women draw up a birth plan. It also includes teaching notes for health professionals.

Handbook for young mothers (Peck, 1990) is an attractive book designed to meet the needs of young mothers.

Section 8: The outcomes of antenatal education

Research into the effectiveness of parent education, in terms of measurable outcomes, has focused largely on the effects of antenatal classes. This is probably as a result of the significance attached to classes *per se* and because it is relatively easy to evaluate the impact of classes which have a discrete start, finish and content (see Appendix 2 for further discussion of this issue).

Recent research studies have set out to measure the impact of parent education on women, in four main areas:

- Their experiences of birth
- Their knowledge
- Their attitudes and feelings
- Their health behaviour

The very small amount of research on the effects on other areas such as women's support networks, perinatal outcomes and experiences of parenting, is also discussed briefly. There are no outcome studies on the effects of parent education on men.

The quality of the research into outcomes of parent education is quite variable (see Appendix 2 for further discussion).

8.1 The experience of birth

Considerable time is taken up in antenatal classes in teaching women techniques and skills which are intended to help them to cope both psychologically and physically with giving birth. The evidence as to whether this works in practice is somewhat contradictory, and seems to vary according to which aspects of birth are measured.

Pain and the use of pain relief

The evidence for a positive effect from classes is clearest here: many authors have reported that women who attend classes experience less pain and use less pain relief than non-attenders (Cogan, 1980, in a review of American research; Bennett *et al.*, 1985). However, two recent studies found no significant differences between attenders and non-attenders (Gunn *et al.*, 1983; Costin and Hurst, 1986). Indeed Costin and Hurst found a reverse trend, with non-attenders rather than attenders experiencing less pain and using less pain relief. They suggest that childbirth preparation can increase anxiety, which in turn may increase the level of pain experienced.

In America, research in the 1980s attempted to assess the effectiveness of different pain-reducing techniques. In one study, relaxation was found to be the most effective component of a pain coping programme (Beck and Siegel, 1980), whilst Geden *et al.* (1985) found sensory transformation (transforming pain into pleasure) to be the only useful technique.

Interestingly, very little attention has been paid to whether women actually use the pain control techniques they have been taught. Some studies assume that women's use of pain relief or their reports of pain, reflect on the use of pain control techniques. Other studies rely on self-reports of the use of pain control techniques. One recent small American study, however, used direct observation of labour, and found that most women did not actually use the breathing or the body positions they had been taught (Lindell and Rossi, 1986). Instead, they moved and breathed in response to individual physiological direction, when encouraged to do so. This study throws into question whether pain control techniques are as useful as health professionals believe. Perhaps, as Lindell (1988) suggests, women have widely differing responses to both pain and pain control techniques and antenatal classes should therefore avoid offering a set prescription of techniques.

Labour length and intervention

An American review of literature suggests that class attendance is associated with shorter labour and few interventions (Cogan, 1980). However, Bennett *et al.* (1985) report that the level of attendance at classes had no effect on labour and labour interventions. Both Costin and Hurst (1986) and Gunn *et al.* (1983) found that class attenders had a longer rather than shorter second stage of labour and more forceps deliveries than non-attenders.

Interestingly, one author has pointed out that the apparently conflicting outcomes of studies on obstetric outcome, can be explained by differences in obstetric management rather than antenatal education (Shearer, 1990). She suggests that the effects of education are swamped by the attitudes and policies of labour and delivery personnel, and therefore recommends evaluating antenatal education purely as education rather than as a tool to change obstetric outcome.

8.2 Improving knowledge

Five British studies in the 1980s assessed women's health knowledge and found significant increases during pregnancy. In three of these studies, knowledge levels were assessed before and after attendance at antenatal classes and increases in knowledge ranged from 10% (Husband, 1983) to 16% (Rutter *et al.* 1988) and 21% (Hillier and Slade, 1989). Interestingly, Husband also followed a group of women who did not attend classes and found a 4% decrease in their knowledge during pregnancy.

Only Hillier and Slade (1989) published their knowledge scale, which is heavily weighted towards knowledge about labour. Three questions covered health during pregnancy: smoking, diet and use of medication. Analysis of changes in knowledge on individual questions showed no significant increases in knowledge for either diet or use of medication, despite the classes covering self-care during pregnancy.

Poor levels of knowledge about diet were also found by Perfrement (1982), who assessed women soon after the antenatal booking visit. She found that 85% of the women had only poor or basic knowledge about diet at this time, but this improved for 26% of the women, when assessed soon after giving birth. The study also notes that those with the worst initial levels of knowledge were the least likely to improve their knowledge of diet.

Four of the studies analyse changes in knowledge by social class and the findings here are contradictory. All report that middle-class women have higher levels of knowledge than working-class women, prior to attending classes. However, Rutter *et al.* (1988) found that working-class women's knowledge increased significantly more than the middle-class women, whilst Husband (1983) and Perfrement (1982) report the reverse trend (though without tests of significance). Hillier and Slade's (1989) study suggests that class attendance eliminates initial social class differences in knowledge.

Hillier and Slade also report that the only factor which can significantly predict the final knowledge level of women attending classes is the individual class attended. They conclude therefore, that the teaching style or personality of the teacher has a strong influence on whether women learn new knowledge, and is much more important than their social class or educational level.

8.3 Influencing attitudes and feelings

In a review of American studies, Lindell (1988) notes that childbirth preparation programmes have been found to promote positive attitudes towards labour and delivery. Findings from recent work in this country are variable. Antenatal classes were found by Rutter *et al.* (1988) to have no effect on the attitudes of mothers and fathers to childbirth, parentcraft classes or hospital care. However, in the Bath study, Taylor (1985) reports that mothers who had attended classes were significantly more likely than non-attenders to have positive attitudes to the staff who cared for them during labour, and not to mind hospital procedures such as shaving or having an enema or episiotomy.

Women's confidence about both labour and childcare may also be promoted through antenatal classes, as reported by Hillier and Slade (1989). The detailed findings of this study are, however, quite complex. Without a control group of women who did not attend classes, it is impossible to know whether women's confidence about labour generally increases during pregnancy irrespective of class attendance. Their finding that confidence levels were unaffected by either the number of classes attended or by dropping out of classes, does suggest this may be so. However, another finding contradicts this somewhat: that the more knowledge a woman has about labour, the more confident she is about labour. This effect was found after classes but not before, and suggests that classes may be as important for validating existing knowledge as for giving new knowledge.

Antenatal education often claims to reduce women's anxiety about pregnancy and particularly labour. Again the evidence is variable with some studies reporting significant reductions in anxiety (for example, Hillier and Slade, 1989) and some finding no effect on anxiety (for example, Lineberger, 1987).

There is some evidence that antenatal education can influence women's emotional and psychological health after the birth. One study suggests that women who attend informal antenatal groups, which provide information about the realities of parenting and which continue to meet postnatally, are less likely to suffer from postnatal depression (Elliott *et al.*, 1988).

8.4 Changing health behaviours

Most health professionals hope to be able to influence health behaviours through education. The behaviours which generally receive most attention are diet, smoking, alcohol and medicine use, breast-feeding and immunization. In all these areas it is hoped to influence behaviour in certain directions which are generally agreed by health professionals to be in the best health interest of the foetus, young baby or the mother herself.

Three recent British studies shed some interesting light on the complex area of behaviour change. Perfrement's (1982) study of women's information during pregnancy found that one third of women improved their diet during pregnancy. Whilst this is an indication of the effectiveness of antenatal education, the author notes that this was only so for some women since 83% were found to have inadequate diets early on in pregnancy.

In Leeds, an intensive programme of antenatal and postnatal visiting with a strong emphasis on health education, achieved improvements in maternal diet, smoking and drinking, with only a small minority of women living in disadvantaged circumstances (Parker and Ness, 1986). The authors report more success in influencing women to immunize their children, with 13% more children completing the full course of immunization in the study group compared with the control group. They conclude that one-to-one health education for women living in an area of social and economic disadvantage needs to be backed up by practical support, such as 'Stop smoking' support groups and the sale of foods not easily or cheaply available in local shops.

In Newcastle a recent project offered increased individual midwifery support to women living in disadvantaged areas who had had low birth-weight babies. The findings of this project are significant since it was carefully designed, and used control groups of women in similar circumstances in order to separate out the effects of the midwifery support. The study demonstrated significant changes in health behaviour for the women who had individual midwifery support (Evans, 1991).

Reductions in smoking were achieved with women who felt least likely to be able to change their behaviour due to the stresses of their social and economic circumstances. More women in the project were also able to change their diet and sustain these changes in the postnatal period than had been able to in their previous pregnancies. The author stresses the significance of the midwives being able to tailor health information and advice to the individual needs and situations of the women concerned through the sustained personal contact they were able to have with the women. This was felt to have been key to the women being enabled to change some of their health behaviours.

Finally, a study from the US is particularly interesting in achieving not only significant changes in smoking behaviour and diet (as a result of one-to-one nutrition counselling and a home-correspondence smoking cessation programme), but also in increasing birth weight (Ershoff *et al.*, 1983).

8.5 Influencing perinatal outcomes

There is no evidence from the literature that antenatal education has any clear effect on perinatal outcomes. Such a direct effect would not be expected given the diversity of factors known to influence low birth weight and perinatal mortality and morbidity.

In a review of American studies, Slager-Earnest *et al.* (1987) report that antenatal education programmes have tended to have little or no impact on infant health. In their own study, however, they found that the babies born to teenagers who had attended a special prenatal education programme had significantly fewer postnatal complications (such as respiratory distress, infections and anomalies) than non-attenders. The authors, whilst noting these findings, caution against attaching much significance to them, since many other variables may have affected such perinatal outcomes.

Two recent British studies suggest that community midwifery practice which involves continuity of care and social support, can have a positive impact of birth weight. Both studies were carefully designed to control a large number of potentially significant variables. The Newcastle project (Evans, 1991) found reductions in low birth weight and pre-term deliveries amongst women involved in the project. The women, who had all had a previous low birth-weight baby received education, care and support which were geared to their individual needs and circumstances. Buckle (1988) reports on a social support intervention by midwives who provided women who had had a previous low birth-weight baby, with support through home visits and telephone calls. The focus for support was broad, and included discussing feelings and anxieties, as well as providing information, advice and referrals to other support agencies. Significant increases in mean birth weights are reported for this study.

These two studies are significant for antenatal education. They suggest that midwifery practice, which is emotionally and socially supportive and offers continuity of care, can contribute significantly to perinatal health outcomes. A part of this includes antenatal education which tackles social and emotional needs and gears information to individual needs and circumstances.

8.6 Building up social support networks

There appears to have been no systematic research to date on the impact of parent education on building up support networks for women.

8.7 A more effective service

Professionals' evaluations of postnatal groups suggest that they may result in parents making more effective and efficient use of health services and the time of health professionals. The following outcomes (unquantified) from postnatal groups are reported:

- Reductions in the number of telephone calls to health visitors about minor problems, and reduced requests for home visits (Tether and Hirst, 1986).
- Saving time for health visitors, since advice given to one member of a group tends to get passed on to others (Labrow, 1986).
- Less health visiting time needed at well baby clinics.
- Less anxiety shown than would normally be expected from first-time mothers (Health Visitor, 1983).
- More appropriate use of child health services (Bracey and Blythe, 1983).
- Parents' seeming to find greater satisfaction in their role as parents (Hiskins, 1982; Bracey and Blythe, 1983).

Two studies also report that mothers who go to postnatal groups tend to experience less isolation and develop more active friendships than other mothers (Hiskins, 1982; Tether and Hirst, 1986). Tether and Hirst found that half of the mothers in their group had had no contact with other mothers prior to the group, and 25% had only met others through antenatal classes. This underlined the importance of the group in fostering support and friendship networks. This was reflected in the finding that *all* the mothers in the group had contact with other group members outside group meetings (58% regularly and 42% occasionally).

8.8 Other outcomes

A number of authors argue against the tradition of evaluating parent education through objective outcome measures. They suggest that process is as important as the outcome, and that parents' subjective evaluation of gains are as significant as measurable objective outcomes (MacKeith and Rowe, 1991). Thus importance is attached to parents feeling more confident, more in control and more able to make choices as a result of parent education (see Section 4.2 for reports of parents' views about the benefits of antenatal classes).

Other authors also argue that if parent education is primarily about education, then what parents have learnt and feel they have gained should be the focus for evaluation (Lindell, 1988).

Section 9: Overview of main findings on parent education

9.1 Antenatal classes

Attendance at classes

Local studies show that only a small minority of women (15–28%) attend a full or nearly full programme of antenatal classes. Class attenders tend to be from middle-class or skilled working-class background, first-time parents, married or in a stable relationship aged 20 or over, and to have average or above average educational attainment. Health professionals are well aware of this situation, and often express great concern that classes are failing to provide education for groups of women who may have a greater need than those who currently tend to attend.

Non-attendance

The main reasons women give for not attending classes are practical difficulties such as transport, childcare and inconvenient times/locations for classes; not knowing about classes; not seeing a need to attend or feeling that they will not be relevant. Health professionals are aware of some of these reasons for non-attendance, and local initiatives such as offering classes in the evening reflect a concern to widen the audience for classes. There is, however, also a common attitude among health professionals that many women have the wrong attitude to their pregnancy or to classes, and that by implication they are to blame for failing to take up what is on offer.

Some women drop out of classes due to giving birth prematurely, the need for early hospitalization or because classes start too late on in the last trimester of pregnancy.

Involvement of fathers and partners

Whilst there is evidence from the literature of increasing concern for the father's role in pregnancy, birth and parenting, few studies have included an evaluation of classes by fathers or partners. Obstacles to involving fathers include: not being invited; not being catered for, except by a special partners' evening or tour of the labour suite; a lack of evening classes to cater for those who work; a low priority being attached to the role and needs of men; a patronizing approach by class teachers.

Fathers in the research carried out for this review, however, expressed a need to talk about hopes and fears for the pregnancy, and for themselves and their partner. They felt that they had fewer opportunities than women to talk about these things, and would have welcomed participation in a group.

The benefits of classes

Both parents and professionals rated classes as beneficial because they provided opportunities for women to learn about pregnancy and labour; to learn techniques of breathing and relaxation; to meet other women and develop support networks. Research into the impact of classes, however, provides conflicting evidence as to whether women use the breathing and relaxation techniques, and whether or not they result in less painful births with fewer interventions necessary. Likewise, research on the impact of classes on women's knowledge is also contradictory. Several studies demonstrate that women from working-class backgrounds know less at the start of classes than middle-class women, and suggest that classes may tend to eliminate these differences. There has been no research on whether classes are successful in building up support networks among women or influencing parenting.

Influencing health

Professionals also rate classes as important in providing an opportunity to influence the health behaviour of women during pregnancy, and how to care for their babies. This is not seen as a primary purpose of the classes by parents, who are in fact critical of the conflicting advice they receive in this area. The few studies which have considered how far classes influence health behaviour have shown that a significant proportion of women may be helped to change their behaviour, for instance, by stopping smoking or altering their diet.

Two areas for improvement suggested by the research are, firstly, to tailor health information and advice much more closely to the social, economic and cultural backgrounds of the individual and, secondly, to provide skills and support for behaviour change in addition to information. Both parents and professionals also express the need for information about health during pregnancy to be covered in the first months of pregnancy, when a woman's behaviour can have the greatest potential impact on the developing baby, rather than later on in pregnancy in antenatal classes.

Parenting and childcare

Health professionals express concern at the need to cover parenting and childcare issues in the antenatal period, but that parents' primary concern is with pregnancy and birth. Parents, however, consistently criticize classes for a lack of teaching about childcare, the role of parents, and the emotional and social aspects of the early months of parenthood.

Other criticisms voiced by parents

Common criticisms voiced by parents in the consumer surveys are: a lack of preparation for labour complications; avoiding or glossing over negative feelings and difficult experiences; an over-emphasis on the baby to the relative exclusion of the mother's needs and experiences; no opportunities to discuss anxieties about body image; finding conflicting advice common and hard to deal with.

Practitioners' dissatisfactions

A number of interlinked dissatisfactions were identified from the literature and from the interviews with professionals. Overall criticisms of classes included: too many needs and issues to cover for the time available; a desire to work with women's agendas but a fear about not covering the professional agenda; how to meet individual needs in a group setting; an over-emphasis on information; fear of tackling negative or difficult issues; insufficient time spent on emotional and social aspects; inappropriate timing of lifestyles advice which was needed earlier in pregnancy.

In relation to teaching methods and resources, the issues were practical difficulties of room and group size inhibiting discussion; how to balance positive and negative experiences; how to use the professionals' own experiences appropriately; a lack of resources and training to run participative group work; an ambivalence over the importance of fostering social contact and support among women; parents' expectations of being given formal talks; a lack of resources of relevance to varying social, cultural, economic, racial and family backgrounds; poor or no access to language interpreters; ambivalence over the use of video and practical difficulties in using it or having access to it; unclear or widely differing aims for parent education; lack of continuity of group membership inhibiting group learning.

Managerial issues

A number of managerial issues were also identified by practitioners which seem to reduce the effectiveness of parent education or inhibit innovation. These included difficulties in getting time in lieu or access to premises for evening work; an unwillingness to try new things because of past failure; rotas preventing continuity of teaching in classes; low or non-existent budgets for purchasing resources, providing refreshments and funding training; a lack of training, updating and peer support; low priority given to the work by managers; concerns about how to evaluate parent education realistically, or evaluation seen as a threat.

9.2 Education within antenatal care

Antenatal care offers ongoing opportunities throughout most of pregnancy for education, support and advice. Since care is taken up by a very large majority of women, it offers the potential for reaching most women, via contact with GPs, midwives and health visitors. This may be the main health service-based educational opportunity for those women who do not go to classes, who tend to have less information and less access to information than those who do go to classes.

The review of research suggests that GPs spend relatively little time on the confirmation of pregnancy visit, and focus largely on medical aspects of pregnancy to the exclusion of social and emotional issues. Rarely do GPs seem to give information on smoking, alcohol or diet, and are not perceived by pregnant women as an important information source. However, GPs have a crucial role to play in information relating to the first 3 or 4 months of pregnancy and particularly for those women who confirm their pregnancy late and then attend the antenatal clinic late.

Throughout antenatal care, pregnant women consistently report a lack of opportunities to ask questions and discuss worries; a lack of privacy for discussion; a lack of staff continuity inhibiting good one-to-one communication; a lack of specific advice and information; or contradictory advice on health issues. The organization of antenatal care, which again is often criticized by women, is also important in influencing the openness of women to education.

There appears to be a lack of co-ordination amongst health professionals about what health issues are tackled, when and by whom, leading to gaps or to repetition. Parents may also be unsure about the role of different health professionals. They may not necessarily see some staff, such as midwives, as qualified to give advice or answer questions, and therefore may not ask questions they wish to have answered.

9.3 The outcomes of antenatal education

There is some research evidence to suggest that antenatal education can influence the knowledge attitudes and health behaviours of pregnant women during pregnancy. For women living in disadvantaged circumstances, antenatal education appears to be most effective when carried out on a one-to-one basis, and when education is geared closely to individuals' circumstances and broader social support is also offered. The impact of an education on labour, delivery and perinatal outcomes is a complex research area in which there is evidence both for and against a positive effect.

9.4 Postnatal education

In the immediate postnatal period in hospital, women tend to find that time for questions and discussion with staff is limited, or not felt to be available. Research with women suggests that they have needs to learn skills relating to the care of their baby, and emotional needs relating to adjusting to their new role. Health staff, however, may have a tendency to focus on problems or care tasks, and not address these wider needs of women.

Parents' use of GPs, child health clinics and visits from health visitors also indicate some mismatch between parents' needs and the ways services are provided. Again, emotional and social needs may be missed out through a focus on medical needs, child development and childcare. There appears to be greater dissatisfaction and less use of these services by both experienced parents and working-class parents. Parents value clinics and health visitors as sources of advice about feeding in particular.

Postnatal groups are not universally available, and are certainly less common than antenatal classes. They vary in the structure, the focus they take and the role that health professionals play. Evaluations of groups by parents suggest that they find most useful a group which is fairly informal and offers them a chance to socialize with other parents, and share experience and problems. Parents also value having informal access to a health professional through a group.

Some research suggests that parents may have unmet needs in the postnatal period relating to postnatal depression, gaining emotional support, problem-solving and opportunities for personal development unrelated to being a parent, but likely to enhance their role as a parent.

The outcomes of postnatal education have been poorly researched. Health professionals identify postnatal groups as a way of reducing their overall workload and enabling them to work more effectively.

9.5 Special provision and special needs

Young parents have special needs arising from their underuse of health services, their increased risks for obstetric and postnatal complications, and a complex of factors related to poor access to housing and income, and experiences of isolation. Teenagers particularly may book late for antenatal care and therefore have less contact with health professionals in the first half of pregnancy. This makes the role of the GP particularly important. Young parents also take up offers of antenatal classes infrequently. Specially targeted classes for young parents are becoming more common, with an emphasis on providing social opportunities, welfare advice and sessions which are informal in nature and largely led by the needs and interests of the group.

Parents from ethnic minority groups also have special needs arising from higher than average rates of obstetric and perinatal complications, low take-up of health services, poorer than average access to housing and employment, experience of racism and, for those whose mother tongue is not English, reduced access to information and communication with health professionals.

Research has highlighted poor access to written information, to antenatal classes and to one-to-one advice and information during pregnancy, for various ethnic minority groups. Although linkworkers are now more available than 10 years ago, some women still appear to experience problems in getting access to a linkworker when one is needed. A large number of local initiatives have recently aimed to increase women's access to maternity services, including parent education. Many of these have focused on teaching pregnant women essential English for pregnancy which, whilst useful, is unlikely to help meet their needs and concerns relating to parent education. There is still a lack of appropriate resources for use with ethnic minority parents.

Although fathers and partners feature in the literature as key people during pregnancy and beyond, their access to education appears to be limited to one or two special sessions within antenatal classes (or much less often, the full set of antenatal classes). In hospital they are seen primarily as supporters of women, and postnatally seem to have little or no access to parent education through groups or an acknowledged role in dealing with child health services. Fathers' needs have been poorly researched and there appears to be some ambivalence within the health service about whether men should be an equal focus for concern to women.

Parents who already have one or more child appear to receive less parent education than first-time parents, both in terms of health professionals' time and in terms of provision such as antenatal classes and postnatal groups. Their needs may include reviewing the previous birth, considering how a new child will fit into the family and updating themselves on health information, hospital procedures and relaxation/breathing exercises. Health professionals also need to improve their information and advice in order to take on board the existing family structure, and to ensure that existing children do not present parents with untoward difficulties in using the services.

Parents with disabilities are largely ignored in the literature. Their special needs may include reduced access to written or verbal information, emotional and social needs arising from their experience of disability, and a lack of support and practical help from health professionals.

Several authors report initiatives to cater for the special needs of women with multiple pregnancies, adoptive parents and parents living in temporary accommodation.

Although working-class women do not generally feature in the literature as a special group, various research studies suggest a similar pattern of lack of access to services and information, and increased risks for obstetric and perinatal complications to young parents and ethnic minority groups. Some studies suggest that the services are geared more to the needs of middle-class women, and that working-class women may perceive and experience pregnancy, childbirth and parenting in quite different ways.

Section 10: Discussion of key issues

This section draws together the main findings of Sections 3–8 and identifies a number of key issues relevant to the development of practice. These are discussed in detail, and provide a basis for the recommendations in Section 11.

10.1 Missed opportunities

Perhaps the most significant issue to emerge from this review is that opportunities for parent education are being missed, and parent education practice is therefore falling short of the expectations and needs of parents. There are five aspects to these missed opportunities.

Needs and provision mismatched

In the antenatal period, there is a marked tendency to equate parent education with antenatal classes. This is evident in two ways. Firstly, in terms of what is actually provided: classes seem to be more generally available to parents than, for instance, adequate time for discussion, questions and information at the antenatal clinic. Secondly, health professionals' perceptions seem to be that antenatal classes are the main forum for parent education, and therefore have become the main focus for training and resourcing.

One consequence of this is that the timing of classes in the last trimester of pregnancy means that earlier needs are missed or met at an inappropriate time. The best example of this is health and lifestyle issues. These are most significant for the health of the mother and baby in the first 3 months of pregnancy, yet continue to be covered in many antenatal classes in the last 3 months. Early pregnancy meetings in some cases are a welcome exception. Not only this, but evidence from research on early antenatal care suggests that many women receive no more than routine advice from their GP in the first 3 months, which is unlikely to be particularly effective in supporting changes in lifestyle.

In the postnatal period, the focus of provision is on one-to-one education and support, with relatively poor provision of postnatal groups. Again, needs and provision are sometimes mismatched, the best example of this being the need for education immediately after the birth. The evidence reviewed in Section 6.1 suggests that the quality of education at this time is often poor and narrow in its focus, leaving women with unmet needs. In recognition of this, health professionals may attempt to cover postnatal needs during the antenatal period in classes. Whilst parents welcome this, the evidence suggests that some aspects such as skill teaching, are best left to the time of need, in the postnatal period.

Certain parents missing out

The focus on classes in the antenatal period is also unsatisfactory because attendance is by no means universal. Low take-up rates mean that in many areas at least half of all pregnant women are missing out on what health professionals see as the main forum for parent education. Classes are not currently a particularly effective way of reaching even the majority of women, and are certainly much worse at reaching fathers. In addition, their take-up by largely White, educated middle-class women means that significant groups of women miss out – particularly women who are young or single or working class or from an ethnic minority group. From evidence reviewed in Sections 3–7, it is clear that these are women who can be considered to be more in need of parent education by virtue of poorer levels of existing information, restricted access to other sources of information, poorer access to health services, and greater chances of ill health for both mother and baby.

Under-estimating education within care

In contrast to antenatal classes, the take-up of antenatal care and of postnatal care in the first few months after the birth, is very high by all groups of women. It provides regular contact with health professionals during a large part of pregnancy, thus offering the potential for ongoing education at the time of need. It may also be the only forum for education for large numbers of women who do not go to antenatal classes or postnatal groups, and who, as detailed above, could be judged to be most 'in need'.

However, the reality seems to be that opportunities for education in care are missed, or are so brief as to be reduced largely to one-way information-giving from health professional to mother. Studies consistently report that significant numbers of mothers feel unable to ask questions of staff, learn very little from their experiences of care, and tend to have their emotional, social and psychological needs disregarded through a focus on medical aspects of antenatal care and baby management aspects of postnatal care.

Focus on women

Women are almost universally the key target group for parent education, despite many authors cataloguing the increasing role of men in childcare and family health. Although antenatal classes may be offered to men in some areas, this is by no means universal, and the research suggests men's needs are not being met. They appear also to be largely excluded from antenatal and postnatal care. To some degree this reflects past splitting of sex roles relating to childcare, but must also be affected by the strong traditions within midwifery and health visiting, of aiming to support, empower and promote the health of women (and through women, the health of children).

A narrow focus for parent education

Much parent education seems to focus on giving information on a narrow range of issues closely related to physical and medical aspects of health during pregnancy and labour and baby management postnatally. Research with parents suggests that social, emotional and psychological needs are being less well recognized by health professionals and less well met both in care and group settings. Current practice therefore seems to meet only certain needs, and largely fails to recognize how social and emotional issues also influence and interact with physical and medical aspects of health.

The emphasis on information in much parent education is also questionable. Whilst education needs an adequate information base, it also needs to encompass attitudes, values and skills in order to be effective.

10.2 Information, education or support?

Through this review, it has become apparent that there is a proliferation of ideas about the aims and purposes of parent education. Some practitioners emphasize the need primarily to support parents, and to do this through working in ways which develop parents' confidence and skills, addressing issues which they identify as relevant to themselves, and encouraging parents to support and learn from one another. In contrast, others emphasize the rights of parents to have health-related information, and the need for health professionals to promote, both overtly and covertly, certain health practices. The emphasis here is often on behavioural outcomes which are seen as beneficial, particularly to the developing baby and child. Both these approaches are claimed to be educational.

Without entering into a lengthy debate about what exactly is meant by education, it is important to try and clarify which approaches might work. The starting point for this must be parents themselves. Parents choose, to a very large degree, how far they make use of antenatal and postnatal services. Their views about what they need and what approaches they find useful are therefore very significant. The review of parents' views in Sections 3–6 are therefore very important. This suggests that parents want the information and support which will help them to make the best choices for themselves and their children. This means providing relevant and realistic information, presenting options and chances to think through these options, and opportunities to consider the experiences of other parents.

This is essentially an open-ended approach which may seem to be in conflict with the health goals of the health service – for example, promoting breast-feeding as in the best health interests of babies. It is, however, pragmatic to recognize that parents cannot, as autonomous adults, be coerced into certain courses of action. An open-ended approach in which health professionals share their knowledge openly and honestly, and support parents to put choices into action, is perhaps the only approach which parents will find acceptable.

This does also raise a difficult issue for the service as a whole – whether parent education can be evaluated in terms of behavioural and health outcomes. Whilst the service as a whole must be evaluated in these terms, at least partially, this may be unrealistic for parent education. Education is only one small part of many factors influencing the behaviour and health of pregnant women and families. The evidence for the effect of structural and material factors such as housing, income and environment on health, is now unequivocal. It is therefore very important that parent educators recognize the limits on what they can realistically achieve. This is particularly so for their work with young parents, working-class parents and those from ethnic minority groups.

A broadly educational goal of meeting parents' learning needs in relation to their experiences of pregnancy and the first months of parenting should therefore be uppermost, whilst not forgetting the broader context of an overall goal for the whole service of health gain.

This is not to deny the research evidence that parent education can lead to health and behaviour changes, as noted in Section 8. It rather suggests that these changes should be one part, albeit a significant part, of the overall aims of parent education, and that the success of parent education should not be judged solely in terms of health and behaviour outcomes. It is also important to remember that the research suggests that a broad approach which includes the emotional and social aspects of becoming a parent and which addresses parents' support needs, is likely to contribute to these goals of health gain and behaviour change.

10.3 Recognizing the interactions between care and education

An important conclusion to be drawn from this review is that there is generally little appreciation of how care and education interact with and influence one another. At the most basic level, formal educational opportunities within care are being missed, as already noted previously. Informal opportunities through the contact women have with one another, are also being missed both antenatally and postnatally.

Perhaps of equal importance is the more subtle effect which the quality and experience of care can have on parents' openness to and expectations of education. Sections 4.1 and 5.5 suggested that professionals providing antenatal care can directly influence the uptake of classes by how much they encourage women to attend. Sections 5 and 6 revealed that many women have needs for asking questions and discussing their pregnancy or their child which are largely unmet along with important social and emotional needs. These needs may be carried over into classes or groups, or may remain unmet by the health services.

Such unmet needs can have several consequences: women lowering their expectations of health professionals, declining to make optimal use of the services, and looking to have these needs met elsewhere. This cycle may then result in women generally rating health professionals poorly as sources of information and support (as noted in Sections 5 and 6). In addition to the issue of unmet needs, aspects of care which are stressful or difficult for parents, will adversely affect their openness to and desire for education through health professionals.

Overall, this has implications for the body of research on parents' views about parent education. Although this research details some criticisms, it is largely favourable, with parents welcoming opportunities for education. It may be, however, that their experiences of care have led to low expectations, that parents are expressing satisfaction only because they have come to expect so little. Without knowing what might be possible, parents are grateful for the *status quo*.

10.4 The need to re-focus parent education

Overall, this review suggests a need to re-focus parent education, both in terms of its content, its target groups, its settings and its timing.

By moving away from a focus on antenatal classes, parents' needs can be addressed more appropriately and more evenly through pregnancy and the early months of parenting. One result of this will be an easing of the pressure on antenatal classes. At present, by being seen as the key opportunity for education, antenatal classes tend to collect a long list of issues to be covered, with different health professionals exerting pressure for their area of concern to be considered. The task for the antenatal teacher who has only six or eight sessions with a group of parents, in sorting out priorities, is unenviable. The pressure to cover so many topics can mean reduced time for discussion, skimming lots of topics, selecting only a few for detailed consideration, or concentrating on basic information needs to the exclusion of other aspects of education such as attitudes and skills. It may also mean that classes are set up to fail by being expected to cover so much in such a short time.

Overall, there is a need for health professionals to place antenatal classes into their proper broad context of the whole range of contact which a woman can have with the health service during pregnancy and the early months of parenthood. Shifting the focus away from classes to the whole of the antenatal and postnatal period should help other opportunities to be used more fully, so that the pressure on classes is reduced and parents' needs can be more appropriately addressed at the time of need. Reduced pressure on classes should also mean that expectations of what they can achieve become less and also more realistic, and this in turn should mean that they are able to become more effective.

Finally, there may also be a need to re-focus antenatal classes themselves. Not only should parents' criticisms of classes be used to shape future work, but there may also be a case for reducing the emphasis currently given to breathing and relaxation. Research into the usefulness of breathing and relaxation techniques, reviewed in Section 8.1, is somewhat inconclusive. Although certain studies do suggest that women perceive there to be benefits, there is also some evidence that techniques may not be used so much in practice and that women can be taught the basic techniques on the labour ward. Perhaps the most useful aspect of these techniques is a psychological preparation for labour. Overall labour is but one small part of the experience of parents, spanning pregnancy, birth and the early months. It is time to reconsider whether it warrants half the time allocation of classes or whether more time could not be better given to some of the social and emotional needs which are currently largely unmet.

10.5 Improving educational quality

The review identified dissatisfaction amongst both parents and professionals with certain aspects of parent education. These relate to its content and the approaches and teaching methods used for both group and one-to-one education. The most common ways suggested for improving quality can be summarized as follows:

- Recognizing the importance of timing parent education appropriately, so that it coincides with parents' specific needs and experiences at the different stages of pregnancy and parenthood
- Recognizing the need to cover feelings, attitudes and skills as well as information
- An equal emphasis on the social and emotional as well as the physical aspects of pregnancy and parenthood
- Tailoring information to the individual needs of parents and ensuring its relevance to their social, economic, cultural and family backgrounds
- Recognizing the limits to personal choice faced by particular groups of parents and designing materials and advice accordingly
- Covering negative feelings and experiences as well as more positive ones

- Using a flexible approach which allows teachers to respond to the interests and needs of particular individuals and groups
- Using participative group teaching methods, which actively engage parents in learning
- Organizing antenatal classes so that they have a fixed start and finish, in order to keep a group together and maximize the effectiveness of participatory group work
- Recognizing the power of parents learning from one another, and finding ways to encourage this, both formally in a group and informally in clinic or class settings
- Using more creative and flexible ways of working with individuals, so that they are more than passive receivers of information
- Recognizing the importance for effective education of parents and professionals building trusting relationships – and therefore the need for continuity of contact.

Interestingly, many of these techniques and approaches are noted to be already in use in some postnatal support groups and in some special antenatal classes. Most notably, many of the classes set up for young pregnant women often encompass many or all of these features. These appear to have developed on the basis of identifying the specific needs of young women, as a result of them rarely attending the usual antenatal classes. Although many of these groups have been running quite successfully for a number of years, there appears to have been little spill-over of ideas and techniques into mainstream antenatal classes.

If educational quality is to be improved in some of the ways outlined above, there will need to be access to training for health professional and suitable resources to support practice. Both, however, appear to lacking.

10.6 A central role for management

The interviews with professionals revealed a complex of interacting factors which amount to parent education lacking managerial support and being given low priority for training, resourcing and development. The chart uses the example of antenatal classes to illustrate how low managerial priority tends to stultify practice and inhibit innovation, which in turn means that take-up rates by parents remain low, which then reinforces the low priority given to the work by managers.

Improvements to the practice of parent education – such as better use of opportunities within antenatal care, and improved education quality – are unlikely to be started or sustained unless there is practical support from health service managers. Attempts to improve practice by changing one or two parts of the equation (such as training in group work skills), are not likely to have much overall impact on practice. They may also result in lower morale and increased cynicism when practitioners' desires to change practice are frustrated by an overall lack of support and resourcing.

It is therefore essential that the future development of parent education practice takes a two-pronged approach, addressing issues of practice alongside and supported by issues relating to management. It is also important at this point

A cyle of low priority/low uptake for antenatal classes

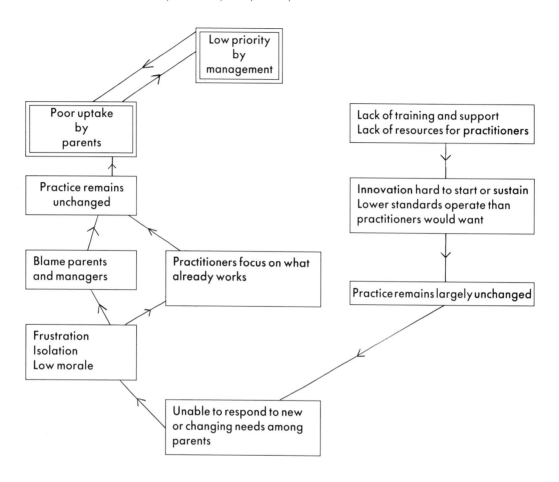

to warn against tackling the managerial issues in isolation from the practice issues and particularly the educational issues. If this happens there may be a tendency for practice to change in ways which make the lives of the service providers easier or more satisfying. These changes, however, may work counter to a better quality of practice for parents. An example of this happening is recent moves in some areas to standardize the order, content and materials used in antenatal classes across a whole district. This appears to happen because managers are recognizing the difficulties practitioners face – difficulties to do with getting hold of resources, lack of planning time, the need to deputize for one another at short notice – and variations in the quality of provision. However, by focusing on solving these problems, there appears to be a somewhat detrimental effect on practice with fixed programmes making it hard or impossible to be flexible enough to meet parents' agendas, and a lack of continuity from the teacher resulting in less effective group work.

10.7 The need to review local practice

In the current climate of health service reorganization and concomitant reviews of priorities, budgets, staffing and professional roles, there is an urgent need for managers and practitioners to review local practice in parent education. This time of change offers opportunities for developing a much clearer rationale for parent education (particularly in relation to outcomes and health gain) and arguing for resource allocation. However, it may also be a time of threat, when parent education comes under scrutiny and may be found to be lacking (for instance, in relation to low take-up rates for antenatal classes). It is therefore essential to the future practice of parent education that both purchasers and providers within and outside health authorities have a clear understanding of the aims and rationale for parent education, and that effective outcomes can be demonstrated.

Local practice therefore needs to be reviewed honestly and critically, with the aim of identifying both effective practice and areas which can be improved. An important aspect to such a review must be the views of parents, who as 'consumers' of parent education are the intended beneficiaries. It is, however, not appropriate to move to a solely consumer-led service in this area of work. There are genuine concerns and issues which the providers of parent education have a professional duty to pursue, whether or not parents say they need or want them. These include using and communicating to best effect their knowledge about maternal and child health, and encouraging parents to use those primary health care services which can help to provide for and protect their health and that of their children. In turn, health professionals involved in parent education also have a duty to communicate the experiences and views of parents about these services, so that they can be developed to meet parents' needs more appropriately. This sets the work of parent education into a much broader context of maternity and primary health care services. Although parent educators are well placed to do this, it appears not to be a particularly significant part of their role at present.

In reviewing local practice, a number of issues are likely to be raised, as practitioners and managers debate appropriate targets for improving practice. A particularly important area for debate is likely to be whether or not to aim for an increase in the take-up of antenatal classes. Although this is an obvious area for improvement, it may prove to be both difficult and expensive to achieve. This review suggests that classes currently cater for and easily attract better-educated middle-class women. Other groups of women tend to see classes as less relevant and often face practical difficulties in attending. If overall take-up rates are to be improved, it is these groups of women which need to be attracted to classes. It is likely that this will involve practitioners not only in changing their practice so that classes are perceived as more relevant, but also in finding ways of enabling women to overcome practical obstacles related to transport, childcare and the need to work. Examples of success in the review suggest that providing a crèche and offering transport may help to improve attendance, along with designing around the needs of a particular target audience. Such efforts can be costly in terms of staff time and resourcing.

An alternative is to look at improving parent education in the antenatal period not through classes but through antenatal care, which already enjoys high levels of uptake. The time and resources involved may be less, and the likelihood of success greater simply because most women are already using this service. This will, however, involve the participation and support of more professionals and requires a willingness of those involved in antenatal care to review practice so that parent education can be maximized. The changes to practice may be relatively small – for instance, ensuring that the occasions for one-to-one health education are appropriate, that there is sufficient time and privacy for it, that women are actively encouraged to ask questions, and that there is as much continuity of care as possible by midwives involved in health education.

A review of local practice will also need to encompass the role of all key professionals, whether or not they recognize themselves as parent educators. Of particular importance is the role of the general practitioner, who is often the only health professional to tackle health education in the first 3 months of pregnancy. Given the constraints on a GP's time at the confirmation of pregnancy visit, it may be that practice nurses with training and expertise in health education are equally well placed to take on this role.

Section 11: Recommendations

11.1 Overall recommendations

Educational quality

The aim of parent education should be primarily educational and therefore not prescriptive about health or behavioural outcomes. There is a need to give equal emphasis to knowledge, skills, feelings and attitudes, and to work to the agendas of both parents and health professionals. Active participation in learning needs to be encouraged so that parents can review their own ideas and knowledge, learn from one another, and apply information to their own circumstances. The information base for parent education needs to develop a greater sensitivity to the individual social, cultural, economic and family backgrounds of parents.

Recognizing individual needs

Parent education needs to develop a greater sensitivity to the individual needs of parents. A particularly important part of this is recognizing the restricted choices which some parents face, and recognizing that for these parents education plays a limited part in enabling change. For parents in poverty or experiencing particular disadvantages, support will be an inextricable part of education. Professionals should be encouraged to recognize how support increases the effectiveness of education, and of how education can itself be supportive through the use of peer learning and an open-ended approach.

A broad focus

Parent education should be relevant to the concerns and lives of parents as they go through pregnancy, labour and the early months of parenting. Greater emphasis needs to be given to the psychological, emotional and social aspects of parents' experiences. A realistic approach means that education should cover difficult as well as positive experiences and issues, and particularly help to create realistic expectations of labour and of parenting. The amount of time generally given to breathing and relaxation in antenatal classes should be reduced in proportion to its significance within the whole experience of becoming a parent, thus releasing time for the consideration of other issues.

Education at the time of need

During pregnancy parents should have opportunities for education at the time of need, appropriate to their stage of pregnancy. Greater emphasis needs to be given to education in the second and especially the first trimester, when the health of the mother can have some influence on the health of the developing baby. Postnatally, more attention could be given to the provision of support groups during the first 6 weeks, and after the first 4 or 5 months.

Maximizing the use of existing opportunities

Many opportunities for parent education go unnoticed or under-used because of a focus of attention on antenatal classes. In practice, many different health professionals are in regular contact with a woman during pregnancy and the early months of parenting, and have a part to play in both education and support. Particular attention should be paid to how routine antenatal and postnatal clinic care can be organized so that parents have more opportunities to ask questions, discuss anxieties and choices, and have more informal contact with other parents who can provide support and share experiences.

In view of the documented fact that the uptake of routine care is far greater than for groups both antenatally and postnatally, priority should be given to increasing the effectiveness of the existing opportunities provided during routine care, rather than attempting to expand the provision of groups. An exception to this is the need for specially targeted antenatal classes for groups considered to either have special needs or reduced access to health services (ethnic minority women and young women in particular). Specially targeted classes for these groups may often provide unique opportunities for education not readily available elsewhere.

Within the health service, recognition is needed of the important part already played by other statutory services and voluntary organizations in parent education.

Fathers and partners

There is an urgent need to consider how parent education can provide for the needs and wishes of fathers and partners. At present, they have virtually no involvement in routine antenatal or postnatal care and only peripheral involvement in postnatal hospital care. Their main access to parent education is through antenatal classes, which are still not generally on offer to all fathers and partners. In the short term, there is a need to extend antenatal class access to as many fathers and partners as possible, and encourage health professionals to consider how, in the longer term, their needs can be met through other health service avenues.

A key role for management

Managers have a central and key role to play in supporting the development of parent education practice. They are in a position to address a number of linked factors to do with staffing, resourcing, training and the status of parent education, which currently stifle the development of practice in many areas.

Managers should take responsibility for reviewing practice in their local area in order to identify barriers to progress, to review targets for improvement, and to support practitioners in the implementation of change. Managers should have the dual aim of firstly improving parents' access to quality parent education, and secondly making parent education a more satisfying area of work for health professionals.

Managers need to develop clear and realistic aims for parent education, and to be able to demonstrate its effectiveness in terms of health gain, changes in knowledge and attitudes, skill development, parental confidence and parental satisfaction.

11.2 Key questions for the development of practice

The following six overall recommendations together amount to a marked shift in the practice of parent education. Because each local area will vary in the ways in which resources and staffing are allocated and managed, it is felt to be inappropriate to conclude this review with a list of very specific recommendations about practice. Instead each health district needs to review its current practice, and identify areas for improvement which take account of their own particular pattern of resourcing and service provision, and the needs of local parents. It would, for instance, be easy to recommend from the literature that special antenatal classes should be set up to cater for young women. However, it could be that in some areas, there already exists good quality antenatal care that is well used by young women, or that many young pregnant women use existing youth or educational services. The most effective use of resources could therefore be to look at ways of improving education within the service the young women already use, rather than setting up something new. This example illustrates well the importance of developing locally appropriate priorities for parent education.

In order to assist readers in beginning this process, there follows a list of key questions which is based on the main findings of this review. These questions highlight important areas of practice which may need to improve. Alongside each question there are a number of examples drawn from the literature, of how practice could be developed in response to the question. These are intended to stimulate thought rather than prescribe certain courses of action.

How can the timing of parent education be made more appropriate to parents' needs?

Examples

- Offer an early pregnancy group meeting, to consider health and lifestyle, choices about place of birth, clinic care and tests
- Teach parenting skills in the early weeks after the birth rather than in antenatal classes.

How can parents' information needs in early pregnancy be better met?

Examples

- Copies of the *Pregnancy Book* (Health Education Authority, 1984) given out by GP clinics
- Encourage GPs to spend longer on the pregnancy confirmation visit and to consider social and emotional aspects of pregnancy as well as medical aspects
- Consider a role for practice nurses in parent education
- Offer an early pregnancy group meeting run by a health professional.

What ways are there of providing support for parents who wish to make changes to their lifestyle?

Examples

- Stop smoking support groups
- Referrals to specialist support agencies.

How can the problem of conflicting advice be reduced?

Examples

- Review or develop district policy on key issues such as dietary advice in pregnancy or infant feeding
- Review the advice in the written literature given to parents
- Consider conflicting advice on an issue itself in antenatal and postnatal groups, and in one-to-one situations, so that parents are better equipped to cope with it.

How can the needs of ethnic minority parents be better met?

Examples

- Linkworkers, interpreters or bilingual health professionals available for group and one-to-one education
- Written information provided in appropriate languages.

What ways are there of giving information which help parents to understand it and apply it to their own lives?

Examples

- Provide information which is relevant to parents in a range of social and economic circumstances
- Avoid prescriptive lists of 'dos and don'ts'
- Encourage parents to talk to other parents in similar circumstances.

How can professionals make better use of many parents' expressed desire to support and learn from other parents?

Examples

- Organize waiting areas and procedures in clinics, hospitals and hospital wards so that parental contact is actively encouraged
- Use participative teaching methods and small group work in antenatal and postnatal groups
- Organize antenatal classes and postnatal groups so that they have continuity of membership, rather than being open to any parents.

Are there ways of integrating education with other services or needs, thus making its take-up easier?

Examples

- Antenatal classes dovetailing with antenatal clinics
- Provide for social needs or practical needs (such as benefit advice) at the same time as antenatal classes
- Integrate parent education into the work of community-based agencies and workers already working with parents (such as nurseries, family centres, adult and community education).

How can antenatal and postnatal care be organized so that there are better opportunities for education?

Examples

- Continuity of contact with staff can help parents to build up a trusting relationship with staff and increase the likelihood of asking for advice and information
- Organize waiting rooms so there is better access to written information, and women are encouraged to talk with and learn from one another
- Explain the support and information health visitors and midwives can offer to parents, who may otherwise not see them as having an educational role.

Are there some fairly simple ways of extending involvement in antenatal classes or postnatal groups?

Examples

- Provide play areas and toys, so that second-time parents are encouraged to attend
- Improve publicity about groups to include written information and reminders.

How can the overall pattern of provision of parent education in groups improve parents' access to education?

Examples

- Have group sessions at various times of day
- Ensure that in areas of disadvantage where parents may face childcare and transport difficulties, local community-based groups are offered
- Actively encourage group parent education in a wide variety of settings, run by a variety of statutory services and voluntary organizations.

How can the views of parents be assessed and used to inform practice?

Examples

- Routine open-ended evaluation of antenatal classes and postnatal support groups by parents
- Periodic small-scale research with particular groups of parents or in particular areas where the uptake of parent education is poor.

How can practitioners be supported to develop their practice?

Examples

- Forum for regular peer support, coordination and updating and coordination of professional activities

- In-service training on participative group work
- Adequate planning and preparation time, and time off in lieu of evening work
- Adequate budgets to support training and the purchase and development of appropriate teaching resources
- In-service training for GPs, health visitors and midwives involved in antenatal and postnatal care on making better use of educational opportunities within care.

11.3 Resources and training

In order to support the development of parent education practice along the lines outlined in the overall recommendations, practitioners and managers will need access to appropriate resources and training. It is therefore recommended that the Health Education Authority consider supporting the following initiatives on training and resource development.

Educational resource for practitioners

A handbook for practitioners is needed which would help people to develop their practice along the lines of broadening the focus for parent education and improving its educational quality (Recommendations 1 and 2). Such a resource would need to include:

- A rationale for parent education
- An overview of approaches to learning
- Effective one-to-one and group work methods
- Practical participatory activities for use in antenatal classes and postnatal groups
- Practical participatory activities and ideas for one-to-one work in care settings

The resource would need to be open-ended and flexible, so that practitioners could use it in response to negotiating agendas with parents. It would also need to provide visual and written stimulus materials of relevance to parents from a variety of social, cultural, educational, economic and family backgrounds. It should provide pointers for how activities and ideas can be adapted to meet individual and group needs, and particularly to encompass the needs of partners and fathers. Given that plenty of information on pregnancy, birth and parenting already exists, its emphasis should be on strategies and activities to help parents review and use such information, and to support one another in their individual experiences.

Overall, such a resource should seek to complement existing resources, aiming to fill gaps rather than replicating existing materials.

Managerial resource for reviewing local provision

Given the need for local practice to develop and change, and given the substantial blocks to such development outlined in this review, managers have a key role to play in supporting local practice. Without their support, parent education practice is unlikely to move ahead significantly. A resource for managers should be developed, in conjunction with the educational resource for practitioners, and cover the following areas:

- How to conduct a review of local practice
- Getting feedback from parents and practitioners about current and future practice
- Setting targets and priorities in relation to the agendas of both health professionals and parents
- Identification of support needs of practitioners
- Support for innovatory practice
- Appropriate outcome and evaluation measures
- Developing a rationale for parent education for both purchasers and providers.

This resource would need to be concise, as practical as possible, and written in such a way as to relate directly to the concerns and priorities of managers in the current climate of Health Service reorganization and change.

Training for practitioners and managers

Given that this review is recommending substantial changes to parent education practice, it will be important to supplement the development of resources with a training initiative. This training should aim to help managers and practitioners review their ideas and practices, and consider how local practice should develop. Overall, the training should be a mechanism for disseminating the two resources, and encouraging them to be used locally as fully as possible.

References

Adams L. (1982) Consumers' views of antenatal education. *Health Education Journal* **41**(1) 12–16.

Artur S. and Butt M. (1991) Post natal exercise and support. *ARM Midwifery Matters* **49**, 13–14.

Association of Community Health Councils in England and Wales (1987) *Antenatal care: still waiting for action*. ACHCEW, London.

Ball J. (1989) Post-natal care and adjustment to motherhood. In: *Midwives, Research and Childbirth*, Volume I, edited by S. Robinson and A. Thomson Chapman and Hall, London.

Beck N. and Siegel L. (1980) Preparation for childbirth and contemporary research on pain, anxiety and stress reduction: a review and critique. *Psychosomatic Medicine* **42**(4) 429–427.

Bennett A. (1985) Antenatal preparation and labor support in relation to birth outcomes. *Birth* **12**(1) 9–16.

Bennett V. (1983) Preparation for parenthood – prenatal care. *Nursing* **2**(19) 567–568.

Billingham K. (1989) 45, Cope Street. *Community Outlook* December, 8–10.

Billingham K. (1990) *Learning Together*. A health resource pack for working with groups. Nottingham DHA Community Unit, Nottingham.

Bishop M. (1988) An introduction to your stay in hospital. *Midwives Chronicle* November, 338–339.

Boyd C. and Sellers L. (1982) *The British Way of Birth*. Pan, London.

Bracey J. and Blythe J. (1983) The post-natal support group. *Community Outlook* March, 70, 75, 77.

Bristol *Evening Post* (1989) Helping out Hartcliffe's young mums. Evening Post, 21 June.

Brown G. (1989) A lone parent group in Yorkshire. *Health Visitor* **62**(6) 187–188.

Buckle S. (1988) Meaningful relationships. *Nursing Times* 12 October, 46–47.

Butler J. (1985) Antenatal classes – are they of benefit? *Midwives Chronicle* **98**(1167) 100.

Campion M J. (1990) *The Baby Challenge*. Routledge, London.

Cartwright A. (1985) What do mothers think about maternity services? *Maternity Action* November/December, 6–7.

Central Statistical Office (1989) *Social Trends* 19 HMSO, London.

Chisholm D.K. (1989) Factors associated with late booking for antenatal care in Central Manchester. *Public Health* **103**(6) 459–466.

Ciliska D. (1983) Early pregnancy classes as a vehicle for lifestyle education and modification. *Canadian Journal of Public Health* **74**(3) 215–217.

Cities Research Unit (1989) *Pregnancy Book Qualitative Research*. Cities Research Unit, London.

Clements J. (1989) Antenatal education. *Nursing Standard* 27 September, 51–54.

Cogan R. (1980) Effects of childbirth preparation. *Clinical Obstetrics and Gynaecology* **23**(1) 1–14.

Conine T. et al. (1986) Provision of preventive maternal health care and childbirth education for disabled women. *Canadian Journal of Public Health* **77**(2) 123–127.

Costin D. and Hurst K. (1986) Time to relax. *Community Outlook* 12 June, 15.

Cox M. (1985) *An Enquiry into Education for Parenthood within the Southend District.* Southend Health Authority, Southend.

Currell R. (1990) The organisation of midwifery care. In: *Antenatal Care. A Research Based Approach*, edited by J. Alexander, V. Levy and S. Roch Macmillan, London.

Curtice L. (1989a) Talking about how difficult we find it. *Health Visitor* **62** 343.

Curtice L. (1989b) *The First Year of Life: Promoting the Health of Babies in the Community.* Maternity Alliance, London.

Curtice L. and Catley J. (1990) Pregnant in Liverpool. *Maternity Action* 46.

Dick-Read G. (1984) *Childbirth Without Fear* (5th edition). Perennial Library, Harper and Row, London.

Dowling S. (1983) *Health for a Change. The provision of preventive health care in pregnancy and early childhood.* Child Poverty Action Group.

Draper J. (1982) The level of preparedness for parenthood. *Journal of Maternal and Child Health* **7**(2) 44, 46–47.

Dunwoody M. and Watters P. (1990) Becoming a mother. *Health Visitor* **63**(10) 335–338.

Early Childhood Development Programme (1987a) The visiting model of the child development programme. Early Childhood Development Programme, Bristol University, Bristol.

Early Childhood Development Programme (1987b) Health visitors and parents: what they think of CDP. Early Childhood Development Programme, Bristol University, Bristol.

Elliott S, Sanjak M. and Leverton T. (1988) Parents' groups in pregnancy: a preventive intervention, for post-natal depression? In: *Marshalling Social Support: Formats, Processes and Effects*, edited by B. Gottlieb, Sage Publications, London.

Ershoff D. (1983) Behavioural, health and cost outcomes of an HMO-based parental health education programme. *Public Health Reports* **98**(6) 536–547.

Evans F. (1991) The Newcastle Community Midwifery Project: the evaluation of the project. In: *Midwives, Research and Childbirth* Volume II, edited by S. Robinson and A.E. Thompson, Chapman and Hall, London.

Evans G. and Parker P. (1985) Preparing teenagers for parenthood. *Midwives Chronicle* September, 239–240.

Fenton P. (1987) Fathers only classes. *New Generation* September, 22.

Field S. (1982) A consumer view of the health visiting service. *Health Visitor* **55**(6) 299–301.

Firdous R. and Bhopal R.S. (1989) Reproductive health of Asian women: a comparative study with hospital and community perspectives. *Public Health* **103**(4) 307–315.

Geden E. (1983) Identifying procedural components for analogue research of labor pain. *Nursing Research* **32**(2) 80–83.

Gillet J. (1985) Preparation for childbirth. *Senior Nurse* 16 March, 8–11.

Gillies E. and Chaudhry M. (1984) Health education sessions on early antenatal and pre-conceptual health: a pilot study. *Health Visitor* **57**(3) 81–2.

Graham H. and McKee L. (1980) *The First Months of Motherhood.* Health Education Council, London.

Green B. and Reavill E. (1989) *PIPSI Activity Pack.* Central Nottinghamshire Health Authority, Nottingham.

Gregory S. (1981) The father's class. *Nursing Times* 29 October, 1894–1897.

Gunn T. (1983) Antenatal education: does it improve the quality of labour and delivery? *New Zealand Medical Journal* **96**(274) 51–53.

Hanson S. and Bozett F. (1986) The changing nature of fatherhood: the nurse and social policy. *Journal of Advanced Nursing* **11**(6) 719–727.

Health Education Authority (1984) *Pregnancy Book*. Health Education Authority, London.

Health Education Authority (1989) *Birth to Five*. Health Education Authority, London.

Health Visitor (1983) A post-natal group for first-time mothers. *Health Visitor* **56** 296–297.

Henderson A. and Brouse A. (1991) The experiences of new fathers during the first three weeks of life. *Journal of Advanced Nursing* **16** 293–298.

Hibbard B. (1989) Antenatal care – past achievements and future needs. *Midwives Chronicle* **102**(1221) 340–343.

Hibbitt E. (1990) Health promotion with homeless families – extending the role of the midwife. *Midwives Chronicle* **103**(1224) 8–10.

Hillier C. and Slade P. (1989) The impact of antenatal classes on knowledge, anxiety and confidence in primaparous women. *Journal of Reproductive and Infant Psychology* **7**(1) 3–13.

Hiskins G. (1982) Personal view. *British Medical Journal* **285**(6336) 204.

Ho E. (1985) Preparing for parenthood. *Nursing Mirror* **161**(3) 14–17.

Holden J. (1990) Emotional problems associated with childbirth. In: *Post-natal care: a research-based approach*, edited by J. Alexande, V. Levy, and S. Roch, Macmillan, London.

Holmes P. (1988) Double trouble? *Nursing Times* 15 June, 16–17.

Husband L. (1983) Antenatal education: its use and effectiveness. *Health Visitor* **56**(11) 409–411.

Hutton E. Having a baby now. *New Generation*, June, 6–7.

Hyde B. (1982) A shared experience. *Nursing Mirror* 4 August, 34–35.

Jackson L. (1990) The happiest time of your life? *Soundbarrier* **43** 10–17.

Jacoby A. (1988) Mothers' views about information and advice in pregnancy and childbirth: findings from a national study. *Midwifery*, **4**(3) 103–110.

Jain C. (1985) *Attitudes of Pregnant Asian Women to Antenatal Care*. West Midlands Regional Health Authority, Birmingham.

Jamieson L. (1986) Education for parenthood. *Nursing* **3**(1) 13–16.

Jeffs J. (1990) Class confidence. *Mother and Baby*, January, 28–29.

Katona C.C.E. (1981) *Approaches to Antenatal Education, Soc. Sc. Med.* Vol. 159, 25–33.

Kelsall J., O'Grady D. and King D. (1990) *Maternity Care for the Deaf*. Wythenshawe Maternity Hospital, South Manchester.

Labrow E. (1986) Self-help postnatal groups. *Health Visitor* **59**(6) 178.

Laryea M. (1989) Midwives' and mothers' perceptions of motherhood. In: *Midwives, Research and Childbirth*, Volume 1, edited by S. Robinson and A. Thomson, Chapman and Hall, London.

Leggett P. (1985) Study of child health clinics. *Health Visitor* **58** 130–131.

Leigh K. (1987) *The Young Parent Club at Wythenshawe Maternity Department*. MIDIRS Information Pack, No. 4, MIDIRS, Bristol.

Lewis V. (1991) *A Good Sign Goes a Long Way. The experience of deaf mothers*. Royal National Institute for the Deaf/Maternity Alliance.

Lindell S. (1988) Education for childbirth: a time for change. *Journal of Obstetrics, Gynaecology and Neonatal Nursing* **17**(2) 108–111.

Lindell S. and Rossi M. (1986) Compliance with childbirth education classes in the second stage of labour. *Birth* **13**(2) 96–99.

Lineberger M. (1987) Pregnant adolescents attending prenatal parent education classes: self-concept, anxiety and depression levels. *Adolescence* **22**(85) 179–193.

Lloyd H. (1990) Getting to know your baby. *Health Visitor* **63**(1) 18–19.

Lloyd P. (1983) Postnatal groups: what format do mothers want? *Health Visitor* **56**(9) 337–338.

Lupton C. (1985) Women's Experience of Antenatal Care. SSRUI Paper No.12. Social Services Research and Intelligence Unit, Portsmouth Polytechnic.

McCabe F., Rocheron Y. and Dickson R. (1985) Antenatal care: a lost opportunity. *Health Education Journal* **44**(1) 51–52.

McCabe F, Rocheron Y, Dickson R. and McCron R. (1984) *Antenatal Education in Primary Care: A survey of general practitioners, midwives and health visitors.* Centre for Mass Communication Research, University of Leicester, Leicester.

McConville A. (1989) Setting up a parenting group. *Health Visitor* **62**(11) 338–339.

McCutcheon M. (1991) *Preparing for the New Life.* Northampton Centre for Health Promotion, Northampton.

Macdonald J. (1987) Prenatal review classes. *Canadian Nurse* October, 27, 29.

McEwan Carty E, Conine T. and Hall L. (1990) Comprehensive health promotion for the pregnant woman who is disabled: the role of the midwife. *Journal of Nurse-Midwifery* **35**(3) 133–141.

McIntosh J. (1988) A consumer view of birth preparation classes: attitudes of a sample of working class primaparae. *Midwives Chronicle* January, 8–9.

McIntosh J. (1989) Models of childbirth and social class: a study of 80 working-class primigravidae. In: *Midwives, Research and Childbirth.* Volume I, edited by S. Robinson and A. Thomson, Chapman and Hall, London.

MacIntyre S. (1981) Expectations and Experiences of First Pregnancy. Occasional Paper 5, University of Aberdeen Institute of Medical Sociology, Aberdeen.

McKee L. (1980) Father and childbirth: just hold my hand. *Health Visitor* **56** 368–372.

MacKeith P. and Rowe A. (1991) Is evaluation a dirty word? *Health Visitor* **64**(9) 292–293.

McKnight A. and Merrett A. (1986) Availability and acceptance of health education among socially 'at risk' pregnant women attending health centres in Belfast. *Family Practice* **3**(2) 85–91.

McKnight A. and Merrett D. (1987a) Alcohol consumption in pregnancy – a health education problem. *Journal Royal College of General Practitioners* **37**(295) 73–76.

McKnight A. and Merrett D. (1987b) Nutrition in pregnancy – a health education problem. *Practitioner* **231** (1427) 530–538.

McRobbie A. (1991) Teenage mothers: a new social state? In: *Feminism and Youth. From Jackie to Just Seventeen.* Macmillan, London.

Macer-Wright (1987) Refreshing parents. *New Generation* March, 22.

Madeley R., Gillies P. et al. (1989) Nottingham Mothers Stop Smoking Project – baseline survey of smoking in pregnancy. *Community Medicine* **11**(2) 124–130.

Mason V. (1989) *Women's Experience of Maternity Care – a survey manual.* Social Survey Division OPCS, HMSO, London.

Maternity Alliance (1985) *Multiracial Initiatives in Maternity Care. A directory of projects for Black and ethnic minority women.* Maternity Alliance, London.

Maternity Alliance (1990) *Your Baby Your Choice. A guide to planning your labour.* Maternity Alliance, London.

Maternity Services Advisory Committee (1982) *Antenatal Care: A guide to good practice and a plan for action.* DHSS, London.

Maternity Services Advisory Committee (1984) *Care During Childbirth.* DHSS, London.

Maternity Services Advisory Committee (1985) *Care of the Mother and Baby (postnatal and neonatal care).* DHSS, London.

Mayall B. and Foster M.C. (1987) Mothers' lament. *Nursing Times* 21 October, 64, 66.

Mayall B. and Foster M.C. (1989) *Child Health Care. Living with children, working for children*. Heinemann, London.

Maybruck P. (1988) Early pregnancy classes. *IJCE* May 17.

Meerabeau L. (1987) Images of fatherhood in antenatal literature: 1. *Health Visitor* **60**(3) 79–81.

Methven R. (1990) *The antenatal booking interview. In: Antenatal care: a research-based approach*, edited by J. Alexander, V. Levy and S. Roch. Macmillan, Basingstoke.

Mills M. (1990) Teenage mothers. In: *Post-natal Care: A Research-based Approach*, edited by J. Alexander, V. Levy and S. Roch, Macmillan, London.

Milner, S. (1990) *Antenatal education: Evaluation report*. Health Promotion and Education Services, Sunderland Health Authority, Sunderland.

Minns H. (1990) Infant feeding in adversity. *Midwives Chronicle* **103**(1224) 3–4.

Moss P. (1986) The first six months after birth: mothers' views of health visitors. *Health Visitor* **59**(3) 71–74.

Munro J. (1988) Parentcraft classes with Bengali mothers. *Health Visitor* **61**(2) 48.

Murphy-Black T. (1986) Evaluation of a Post-basic Training Course for Teachers. Unpublished PhD thesis, University of Manchester.

Murphy-Black T. and Faulkner A. (1988) *Antenatal Group Skills Training. A manual of guidelines*. John Wiley.

National Childbirth Trust (1991) *NCT Teachers Annual Returns 1990: Outreach*. National Childbirth Trust, London.

NCOPF (1979) *Pregnant at school*. Joint Working Party on Pregnant Schoolgirls and Schoolgirl Mothers, National Council for One ParentFamilies Community Development Trust.

Newham Parents Forum (1988) *A Treasured Experience? What women said about Newham Maternity Hospital*. Newham Parents Forum, London.

Nunnerley R. (1985) Teenage dilemma. *Midwives Chronicle* **98**(1172) 244–248.

OPCS (1991) *Birth Statistics VS2, 1990*. OPCS, HMSO, London.

Parker M. and Ness M. (1986) Supporting city mothers. *Community Outlook* 18 October, 20–21, 23.

Pearson M. (1985) *Racial Equality and Good Practice Maternity Care*. Training in Health and RaceCentre for Ethnic Minorities Health Studies. Health Education Council and National Extension College, London.

Pearson J. and O'Brien M. (1987) Reach out and touch the fathers in your classes. *New Generation*, June, 19–20.

Peck F. (1990) *Handbook for Young Mothers*. Rainer Foundation.

Perfrement S. (1982) *Women's Information on Pregnancy, Childbirth and Babycare*. Centre for Medical Research, University of Sussex, Brighton.

Perfrement S. (1984) New ideas for mothers and midwives. *Nursing Mirror*, Vol. 158, No. 14.

Perkins E. (1979) Defining the need: an analysis of varying teaching goals in antenatal classes. *International Journal of Nursing Studies* **16** 275–282.

Perkins E. (1980) The pattern of women's attendance at antenatal classes: Is this good enough? *Health Education Journal* **39**(1) 3–9.

Perkins E. and Morris B. (1981) Should we prepare for parenthood? *Health Education Journal* **40**(4) 107–110.

Phoenix A. (1991) *Young Mothers*? Polity Press, Cambridge.

Porter M. and MacIntyre S. (1989) Psychosocial effectiveness of antenatal and postnatal care. In: *Midwives Research and Childbirth*, Volume 1, edited by S. Robinson and A. Thomson A, Chapman and Hall, London.

Precey G. (1986) *Early Pregnancy Classes*. Maternity Alliance, London no. 24, p.9.

Priest J. and Shott J. (1991) *Leading Antenatal Classes. A practical guide.* Butterworth Heinemann, Oxford.

Prince J. and Adams M. (1990) The psychology of pregnancy. In: *Antenatal Care. A research-based approach*, edited by J. Alexander, V. Levy and S. Rochm Macmillan, London.

Redbridge and Waltham Forest Area Health Education Service (1980) *Education in the antenatal period*. Redbridge and Waltham Forest Area Health Authority.

Rees C. (1982a) Antenatal classes: time for a new approach. *Nursing Times* 25 August, 1446–8.

Rees C. (1982b) *What Did We Learn? An assessment of an antenatal education group skills workshop*. South Glamorgan Health, Authority, Health Promotion Unit.

Robertson A. (1988) *Teaching Active Birth*. Ace Graphics.

Rocheron Y. and Dickinson R. (1990) The Asian mother and baby campaign: a way forward in health promotion for Asian women. *Health Education Journal* **49**(3) 128–133.

Rotheram J. (1989) Care of the disabled woman during pregnancy. *Nursing Standard* 29 November, 36–39.

Ruel A. and Adams G. (1981) A parenting group in general practice. *Journal of the Royal College of General Practitioners* **31** 496–499.

Russell K. (1988) Early teenage pregnancy. *Maternal and Child Health* **13**(2) 43–46.

Rutter D., Quine L. and Hayward R. (1988) Satisfaction with maternity care: psychosocial factors in pregnancy outcome. *Journal of Reproductive and Infant Psychology* **6**(4) 261–269.

Sadler C. (1988) The generation game. *Community Outlook* July, 20–22.

Sefi S. (1987) Running a post-natal exercise group. *Health Visitor* **60**(6) 197.

Shearer M. (1990) Effects of prenatal education depend on the attitudes and practices of obstetric caregivers. *Birth* **17**(2) 73–74.

Sherratt F., Johnson A. and Holmes S. (1991) Responding to parental concerns at the six-month stage. *Health Visitor* **64**(3) 84–86.

Simms M. and Smith C. (1984a) Teenage mothers: later attenders at medical and antenatal care. *Midwife, Health Visitor and Community Nurse* **20**(6) 192, 196–197, 200.

Simms M. and Smith C. (1984b) Teenage mothers: some views on health visitors. *Health Visitor* **57**(9) 269–270.

Simms M. and Smith C. (1986) *Teenage Mothers and Their Partners. A Survey in England and Wales*. Department of Health and Social Security, HMSO, London.

Slager-Earnest S., Hoffman S. and Anerson Beckmann C. (1987) Effects of a specialised prenatal adolescent program on maternal and infant outcomes. *Journal of Obstetrics, Gynaecology and Neonatal Nursing* **16**(6) 422–429.

Smith J. and Whitehead N. (1986) Postnatal support: what do mothers want? *Health Visitor* **59**(6) 174–176.

Spillman J. (1990) Multiple births – parents' anxieties and the realities. In: *Antenatal Care. A research-based approach*, edited by J. Alexander, V. Levy and S. Roch, Macmillan, London.

St. Clair P and Anderson N. (1989) Social network advice during pregnancy: myths, misinformation and sound counsel. *Birth* **16**(3) 103–108.

Staines C. (1983) Preparation for parenthood. *Nursing* **2**(19) 565–566.

Stewart A. and Ring W. (1991) What about adopters? *Health Visitor* **64**(9) 297–299.

Stocks V. (1982) Are they worth reading? *Mother and Baby* April, 12–14.

Stringer E. (1986) Pregnant teenagers group. *Maternity Action* **23**, 9.

Taubenheim A., and Silbernagel T. (1988) Meeting the needs of expectant fathers. *Professional Nurse* **3**(10) 378.

Taylor A. (1985) Antenatal classes and the consumer: mothers' and fathers' views. *Health Education Journal* **44**(2) 79–82.

Taylor A. (1986) Maternity services: the consumer's view. *Journal of the Royal College of General Practitioners* **36**(285) 157–160.

Tether M. and Hirst S. (1986) Postnatal support group. *Health Visitor* **59**(6) 178–179.

Tew M. (1990) *Safer Childbirth? A Critical History of Maternity Care*. Chapman and Hall, London.

Thompson H. (1982) What about father? *Community Outlook* 14 April, 99–100, 103–104.

Todd J. (1988) Teenage club at the Royal Berkshire. *Midwives Chronicle* **101**(1207) 238.

Townsend P. and Davidson N. (1982) *Inequalities in Health: The Black Report*. Penguin, London.

Two Can Project (1984) *Relaxation Classes*. Two Can Project, Derby City Hospital.

Watson G. (1991) Cherishing the pregnant teenager. *Midwife, Health Visitor and Community Nurse* **27**(4) 114, 116.

Webber A. and Janzen R. (1982) Antenatal education – does it work? *Midwives Chronicle* March, 94–97.

Whitehead M. (1987) *The Health Divide: Inequalities in health in the 1980s*. Health EducationCouncil, London.

Williams M. and Booth D. (1985) *Antenatal Education. Guidelines for teachers*. Churchill Livingstone, Edinburgh.

Willis A. (1988) Working with fathers in the inner city. *Social Work Today* 19 February, 12–13.

Wilson A. (1986) With a little help from your friends. *Parents* December, 87–88.

Wilson P. (1990) *Antenatal Teaching. A guide to theory and practice*. Faber and Faber, London.

Woollett A. and Dosanjh-Matwala N. (1990a) Asian women's experiences of childbirth in East London: the support of fathers and female relatives. *Journal of Reproductive and Infant Psychology* **8**(1) 11–22.

Woollett A. and Dosanjh-Matwala N. (1990b) Pregnancy and antenatal care: the attitudes and experiences of Asian women. *Child Care, Health and Development* **16**(1) 63–78.

Appendix 1: Professionals interviewed for the review

Kate Billingham   Development Officer for Health Visiting, Nottingham Health Authority
Mary Bonomaully   Health Visitor, Saffron Group Practice, Saffron Lane, Leicester
Hazel Brewer   Health Visitor, Saffron Group Practice, Saffron Lane, Leicester
Marietta Evans   Health Promotion Officer, Sunderland Health Authority
Melanie Every   Professional Officer, Royal College of Midwives
John Goodchild   Exploring Parenthood
Chris Gowdridge   General Secretary, Maternity Alliance
Barbara Green   Health Visitor, Kirklington Road Surgery, Rainworth, Nottinghamshire
Lizzie Hibbitt   Parentcraft Coordinator, St Mary's Hospital, Paddington
Debbie Jackson   Health Promotion Officer, Halton Health Authority
Helen Lewison   National Childbirth Trust
Sylvia McGuiness   Chair of Teachers' Panel, National Childbirth Trust
Pippa McKeith   Team Leader, 45 Cope Street, Nottingham
Ros Meek   Professional Officer, Health Visitors Association
Rosemary Phillipson   Health Visitor and Midwife, 45 Cope Street, Nottingham
Maureen Short   Health Visitor, Hylton Castle Health Centre, Sunderland
Tricia Vinycomb   Coordinator, Wessex Parent Education Project
Jen Young   Community Midwife, Hylton Castle Health Centre, Sunderland

The groups of health visitors and midwives attending discussions at Birmingham Maternity Hospital and Halton General Hospital in June 1991.

Appendix 2: A discussion of the research evidence used in this review

In collecting together the literature for this review, more than half of the articles identified by a computer search on antenatal and postnatal education were about antenatal classes. Likewise the large majority of the outcome studies focused on measurable outcomes of classes. This dominance of classes within the literature has several drawbacks. Firstly, it reinforces the equating of antenatal education with classes, as already noted in the review. This means that classes are rarely set within the whole context of the antenatal period. When it comes to evaluating classes, this is a significant drawback to many of the studies which tend to ascribe measurable outcomes to classes without considering the many other factors which may influence women's knowledge and behaviour during pregnancy. Secondly, since only a minority of women attend classes, and since these tend to be more middle-class and better educated women (see Section 4) evaluation of classes is not a very reliable indicator of whether parent education works and certainly is not likely to be representative of parents as a whole.

This focus on researching classes may partly be because it is easier to investigate their effects than education within the whole antenatal period. Classes have a definite start and finish and therefore allow pre- and post-class measurements to be made. However, despite this, many of the studies of classes have a number of significant weaknesses. None of these reported are able to ascribe cause and effect: they simply report changes that happen to pregnant women over a period of time during which they attend antenatal classes. A few studies are on stronger ground by having control groups who did not attend classes, but overall, there is little acknowledgement of or attempt to take account the range of factors which might influence women's education about pregnancy, childbirth and parenting. Again, the studies of outcomes from antenatal classes reported in Section 8 generally fail to distinguish frequency of attendance or to give details of the content or variety of sessions either on offer or attended by the women being studied. The studies therefore offer very few clues as to which aspects of parent education are working, or not, and for which groups of women.

The timing of surveys with women on their views of classes is also an important variable. Some surveys asked women for their views immediately after the classes ended but before birth, some immediately after delivery and others at least one month after birth. Memories of the classes are therefore likely to vary considerably, but more importantly, parents' own experiences of giving birth and of the early months of parenthood will affect how they rate the classes. If one of the aims of classes is to prepare parents for birth, then it is less informative to ask for their views of classes before the birth compared with after the birth. Similarly, if classes are also intended to help prepare parents for the early months of parenthood, it is important that surveys assess parents' satisfaction with classes several months after the birth rather than in the immediate postnatal period. There are, however, no research surveys which fulfil these criteria.

Appendix 3: Research methods, recruitment, design, definitions, selection criteria and characteristics of the groups in the research

Recruitment and methods

Parents were recruited to the groups through an independent fieldwork agency. The agency was instructed not to recruit women via health services such as clinics or health centres, in order to avoid a bias towards women who used the services, or any association between the discussion groups and the health services. The fieldwork agency undertook to recruit people to the groups on the basis of agreed criteria. Quotas were set for the groups to ensure variation on the key criteria of age, ethnic origin, marital status and socio-economic group.

A total of 44 women took part in seven different discussion groups in the West Midlands. Of these 21 were 26 or more weeks pregnant, 16 for the first time, and 5 (all in one group) for the second time. The remaining 23 women each had a first baby, aged up to 9 months. Two additional groups were run, one for fathers and prospective fathers and the second for Asian women who were currently pregnant and/or had at least one child. All but one of the Asian women taking part spoke some English and the discussion took place in English with some translation by group members for one another. The Asian women were of Bangladeshi and Mirpur Pakistani origins. Table 5 shows the overall characteristics of the parents taking part in the research (see p. 133 for a separate breakdown for pregnant women and first-time mothers).

Groups for pregnant women were run separately from the groups for new parents so that people's experiences in these two periods could be distinguished. Two exceptions to this were the fathers group and the Asian group, where prospective parents and new parents met together, since there were insufficient resources to run two separate groups for each. Table 6 shows the locations and timings of the different discussion groups.

Table 5: Characteristics of parents in the research

Socio-economic groups		Age		Marital status	
ABC1	29%	18–24	43%	Single	24%
C2DE	64%	25–29	45%	Married or co-habiting	76%
Unemployed and not classifiable	7%				

Race		Location		Antenatal class attendance	
Caucasian	64%	Urban	36%	Non-attenders	57%
Asian	14%	Suburban	29%	Attenders	43%
Afro-Caribbean	22%	Rural	35%		

Table 6: Locations and timings for the discussion groups

Rural		Suburban		Urban	
Pregnant women	evening	Pregnant women	afternoon	Pregnant women	morning
New mothers	afternoon	New mothers	morning	New mothers	morning
Fathers and prospective fathers	evening	Second-time mothers (pregnant)	afternoon	Asian pregnant women and new mothers	afternoon

Discussion groups were held in the homes of the fieldwork recruiters or local community centres. They lasted about 1.5 hours and were tape-recorded with the permission of the group. It was made clear that if quotes were used they would be anonymous. Babies were welcomed to the groups and each session began informally with refreshments. A small payment was made to those taking part, and where necessary, taxi or bus fares reimbursed.

At the start of each group session, the researcher explained the purpose of the work, and took care to emphasize two points: firstly, that she was independent, not employed by the health service and had no contact with staff in the area; and secondly, that the group session was an opportunity for parents to have a say about their experiences and how they felt about the health services on offer. It was hoped that this would give parents the freedom to talk openly and honestly, without fear of repercussions, and with the clear purpose of giving feedback to health professionals.

A series of open-ended stimulus questions was used to promote group discussion. At times, key points were recorded on large sheets of paper, as a way of reinforcing the importance attached to the parents' experiences and views. Transcripts of the group sessions were analysed in order to identify common issues and themes across the different groups.

Research design

In deciding on the research design for the discussion groups at the outset, there were three variables which were felt to be particularly significant: location; socio-economic group; and parent status. Firstly, three locations were felt to be important (rural, suburban and urban) because of a likely influence on access to health services. Secondly, a split into two socio-economic groupings, ABC1 and C2DE, was also felt to be desirable, because of likely differences in the ways people would contribute to discussion groups and differences in access to both health services and resources for pregnancy and parenting. Thirdly, it was important not to mix pregnant women with those who already had a baby in order to allow their needs and experiences to be identified separately. It was not, however, possible within the resources available, to plan groups to take full account of these three key variables. The design for groups shown in Table 4 therefore represents a compromise, in which pregnancy/parent status is the main variable.

Other variables which were considered but felt to be of relatively less significance were age, attendance at antenatal classes and marital status. These factors were, however, considered in relation to the quotas for each group.

Definitions used in the research

- Pregnant woman: at least 26 weeks pregnant and has not had a live birth (excludes early childhood death or cot death; includes those with existing step-child(ren) or who have previously had miscarriage or stillbirth and are currently pregnant)
- First-time mother: has a child aged up to 9 months and this is the first child (excludes those with one child now, but another lost through early childhood death or cot death; includes those with one child now and another lost through stillbirth)
- Attender at antenatal class: has attended at least three sessions, or attended twice and intends to continue attending
- Non-attender at antenatal class: has attended one or no sessions and has no intention of attending in future
- Second-time mother: has had one child born alive and is currently 26 weeks or more pregnant with second child.
- Fathers and prospective fathers: partner of pregnant woman or first-time mother (as defined above), but not of any woman taking part in any other group
- Socio-economic group: using Registrar General's classification of occupations for male head of household

Selection criteria for groups

The following criteria were used for recruitment to a group of ten people.

Age

18–24: 5 people
25–29: 3 or 4 people
30+:   1 or 2 people

Note 1: Age criteria were based on the proportions of first-time live births to different age groups, in England and Wales in 1988 (unpublished figures supplied by the Fertility Statistics Unit at the Office of Population Censuses and Surveys, London).

Note 2: Women under the age of 18 were excluded from this research. It had originally been intended to run a special group for pregnant women under the age of 18, but recruitment difficulties led to this being shelved.

Marital status

Single: 2 people
Married/cohabiting 8 people

Note 1: In 1987, 24.8% of all births were registered as occurring outside of marriage. Of these 68% are reported as being registered by both parents and of these 70% gave the same address (Central Statistical Office, 1989). This implies that overall, 48% of births outside marriage were to cohabiting couples (and therefore account for 11.9% of all births). The remaining 12.9% of births outside of marriage are therefore likely to be to single women. There are no published figures on first-time births outside of marriage.

Note 2: For the selection criteria, it was felt to be more important to have two single mothers per group in order for them to feel comfortable, than to reflect the national statistics (12.9 births to single parents).

Ethnic group

Rural and suburban: 8 White
                    2 Asian or Afro-Caribbean
Urban: 6 Asian or Afro-Caribbean
                    4 White

Note: Recruitment of Asian and Afro-Caribbean people in the rural and suburban locations proved very difficult, with only 2 out of 26 non-Caucasian people being recruited to these groups. In the urban groups, 9 out of 13 women were Afro-Caribbean. A further 8 Asian women took part in an additional group.

Antenatal class attendance

Minimum of 3 attenders and 3 non-attenders
Note: For the sample overall, and for the pregnant women and first-time mother groups, attendance rates at antenatal classes fell within these limits. However, it proved impossible to meet these criteria for each group. In the urban locations, all the women were non-attenders (except for two women in the Asian group), whilst in the rural locations 75% were attenders.

For additional groups: socio-economic group – a mix of ABC1 and C2DE groups, as far as possible.

For first-time mothers: a minimum of six with a child aged 0–5 months.

For fathers and prospective fathers: age and antenatal class attendance based on partner rather than father.

Characteristics of the groups

Pregnant women and first-time mothers

Characteristics		Pregnant women	First-time mothers
Socio-economic group	ABC1	31%	33%
	C2DE	69%	66%
Age	18–24	50%	54%
	25–29	50%	25%
	30+	–	21%
Marital status	Single	25%	38%
	Married/cohabiting	75%	62%
Ethnic group	Asian	–	–
	Caucasian	75%	71%
Attendance at	Non-attender	69%	58%
antenatal classes	Attender	31%	42%
Total number participating		16	23

First-time mothers: all babies were aged 0–5 months, except for two who were aged 6–9 months.

Additional groups

Characteristics		Second-time mothers	Asian women	Fathers and prospective fathers
Socio-economic group:				
ABC1		3	–	1
C2DE		2	4	5
Unemployed		–	4	–
Age	18–24	–	3	1*
	25–29	5	3	4
	30+	–	2	1
Marital status				
Single		–	–	1
Married/cohabiting		5	8	5
Ethnic group				
Asian		–	8	–
Afro-Caribbean		2	–	–
Caucasian		3	–	6
Attendance at antenatal classes				
Non-attender		3	2	4*
Attender		2	6	2
Stage of pregnancy				
Less than 26 weeks		–	3	–
More than 26 weeks		5	5	6
Number of other children				
	0		–	1
	1	5	5	2
	2		–	4
	3		–	1
Total number participating		5	8	6

*Refers to partner's age and attendance at classes, and not that of the father.